Prentice Hall Health

question and answer review

for the Pharmacy Technician

Marvin M. Stoogenke, R.Ph.
Mercy Medical Center
Baltimore, Maryland
President, Pharma-Tech Training, Inc.

Peter Le, R.Ph., MBA
Director of Pharmacy
Leland Medical Plaza
Garland, Texas

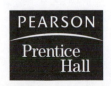

PEARSON

Prentice
Hall

Upper Saddle River, New Jersey 07458

Library of Congress Cataloging-in-Publication Data

A CIP catalog record for this book can be obtained from the Library of Congress.

Publisher: Julie Levin Alexander
Assistant to Publisher: Regina Bruno
Acquisitions Editor: Mark Cohen
Associate Editor: Melissa Kerian
Editorial Assistant: Mary Ellen Ruitenberg
Marketing Manager: Nicole Benson
Channel Marketing Manager: Rachele Strober
Director of Production and Manufacturing:
    Bruce Johnson
Managing Production Editor: Patrick Walsh
Production Liaison: Alexander Ivchenko

Production Editor: Jessica Balch, Pine Tree Composition
Manufacturing Manager: Ilene Sanford
Manufacturing Buyer: Pat Brown
Design Director: Cheryl Asherman
Design Coordinator: Maria Guglielmo Walsh
Cover and Interior Designer: Janice Bielawa
Composition: Pine Tree Composition, Inc.
Manager of Media Production: Amy Peltier
New Media Project Manager: Stephen Hartner
Printing and Binding: Banta Book Group
Cover Printer: Phoenix Color Corp.

Pearson Education, Ltd., *London*
Pearson Education Australia Pty. Limited, *Sydney*
Pearson Education Singapore Pte. Ltd.
Pearson Education North Asia Ltd., *Hong Kong*
Pearson Education Canada, Ltd., *Toronto*
Pearson Educación de Mexico, S.A. de C.V.
Pearson Education—Japan, *Tokyo*
Pearson Education Malaysia, Pte. Ltd.
Pearson Education, Upper Saddle River, New Jersey

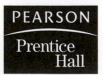

10 9 8 7 6 5 4 3 2
ISBN 0-13-041650-9

Contents

Preface / v
Acknowledgments / ix
Introduction / xi

1 Assisting the Pharmacist in Serving Patient Medications / 1
2 Mathematical and Pharmaceutical Calculations / 89
3 Pharmacy and Medical Terminology / 124
4 Dispensing Process and Information Resources / 148
5 Medication Distribution and Inventory System / 187
6 Management of Facilities, Resources, Information, and Understanding
   of the Laws Relating to Pharmacy / 195

Index / 219

Preface

INTRODUCTION

Health care is dynamic. Pharmacy as part of this dynamic environment is in constant evolution. Changes mean new roles for the current cast and openings for new cast members. Although pharmacy technicians have been practicing for some time, until now their role was rudimentary. The traditional pharmacy technician supported distributive services under the supervision of a pharmacist by performing simple tasks. These included filling the prescription with the appropriate drug, packaging the medication in the proper container, and affixing the label containing the directions for use as intended by the prescriber. Pharmacy practice, regardless of the setting, was basic and the pharmacy technician's role was, likewise, basic. The fundamental tenet guiding the pharmacy technician has been to provide the right drug to the right patient at the right time.

As health-care delivery changes to accommodate the needs and wants of patients, legislative mandates, technology, and much more, the services associated with pharmacy practice also change. Pharmacists who practice only distributive pharmacy are recognizing that they must expand their roles to include providing information to patients and to other health-care professionals. In addition, pharmacists have a more significant role in other non-distributive pharmacy practices such as cost containment, formulary services, and third-party payers. The pharmacy technician closes the potential gap in traditional pharmacy delivery that these major changes in health care are creating. However, in order to continue to deliver the traditional services of pharmacy without interruption in patient care, pharmacy technicians must be qualified by having the proper knowledge, appropriate skills, and competence to provide these services.

In order to assure the smooth operation of distributive pharmacy, the Pharmacy Technician Certification Board certification program was developed to assist in defining the role of pharmacy technicians. Certification is a significant career progression that establishes uniformity of knowledge, consistency in applying that knowledge, and the basis for a standard of practice. The National Pharmacy Technician Certification Examination is a formal vehicle by which pharmacy technicians are determined to be qualified to perform the tasks associated with distributive pharmacy practice.

The author designed this text to assist the reader in studying for and successfully completing the National Pharmacy Technician Certification Examination. In addition, this review guide is a valuable tool for students in on-the-job training programs or informalized pharmacy technician training programs. It can be used in conjunction with a pharmacy textbook such as *The Pharmacy Technician,* a drug handbook such as the *Drug Information Handbook,* and a medical dictionary. The questions are comprehensive, easily read, and aligned with the national examination. As an enhancement to the learning experience, many questions were derived from actual pharmacy events.

The qualified pharmacy technician applies the principles of accurate and safe pharmacy practice. This is accomplished through knowledge of drug names and uses, medical and pharmacy terminology and abbreviations, calculations, laws regulating practice, and common disease states, symptoms, and the medications used to treat them. The pharmacy technician's responsibilities and activities are governed by standards of ethics. These standards direct the pharmacy technician in the selection of the appropriate drug, correct strength and form, and the preparation of understandable label directions for the patient or caregiver.

This review book tests the extent of knowledge required to do the job while assuring that the patient's safety and well-being are primary. The author has tried to correlate principles derived from pharmacy ethics with the information required for the certification examination. Certification is a means of establishing credibility. Certification is the first step.

OVERVIEW

Question and Answer Review for the Pharmacy Technician is a basic review guide to help you structure your study for the national certification examination and to assist you with classroom work or on-the-job training programs. This review book contains an abundance of questions to prepare you for taking tests. The questions are constructed to assist you in studying for each section of the certification examination for pharmacy technicians.

The National Pharmacy Technician Certification Examination is used to test the qualifications of individuals working in a pharmacy setting who work under the supervision of a licensed pharmacist. The role, duties, and responsibilities of the pharmacy technician are supportive. The pharmacy technician assists the pharmacist in delivering services. Hence, the examination focuses predominantly on the area of "Assisting the Pharmacist in Serving Patients." This area of the examination is worth 64% of the total score. It focuses on traditional distributive pharmacy activities that involve the processing of drug orders. The pharmacy technician's job includes receiving the drug request by prescription (traditionally used in the outpatient setting) or medication order (typically found in the inpatient or institutional setting). Competence is measured by the ability to process new orders or refills received in various formats (hardcopy or electronic) as well as thoroughness in assessing authenticity and patient information regarding allergies, sensitivities, previous adverse reactions, and illness.

Questions test the candidate's knowledge of products, calculations, conversions, and terminology. (*Note:* drug products are indicated by brand or trade names in capital letters and generic names in lower case letters). Various specifics within pharmacy practice are covered and include compounding, intravenous admixture preparation, packaging, labeling, and various types of record keeping.

The second area of the examination deals with "Maintaining Medication and Inventory Control Systems." This section contributes 25% to the overall test. Activities in this section include the handling of drugs to assure their availability. Pharmacy technicians are expected to understand the purchasing process, inventory control, and stocking in accordance with approved job-centered policies and procedures. The candidate should be aware of the way orders to vendors are placed, the activities initiated when goods are received, and the controls which assure orders can be filled using available stock without exceeding the pharmacy's budget. The pharmacy technician should note that stock in many cases includes more than drugs. Stock may also include durable medical equipment inventory, devices, and supplies.

The third and final area of concentration, "Operations," includes administrative functions pertinent to pharmacy operations. These include human resources, facilities and equipment maintenance, communications, policies and procedures, compliance with regulations and professional standards, and the use of computer systems. This section is 11% of the overall test.

Studying this review text in conjunction with the author's textbook, *The Pharmacy Technician,* a drug handbook, and a medical dictionary should provide abundant information covering each area of the examination. Preparation, as well as a good night's rest, is essential to successful completion of the examination.

NOTE FROM THE AUTHOR

As a pharmacist, I have been associated with pharmacy technicians for many years. As an author, I have provided a basis for anyone interested in becoming a pharmacy technician to learn a uniform body of knowledge in a practical manner. My experiences have been gratifying. Pharmacy technicians have often impressed me with their know-how and enthusiasm.

The future for pharmacy technicians is bright and full of opportunities. The changes continuously occurring in health-care delivery will benefit the pharmacy technician's career prospects. Only now are we noticing the importance of the technician on a global scale. The pharmacy technician will play a key role in keeping distributive pharmacy alive and pharmacy costs in line with the mandate for prudent health-care economics.

You are at an ideal point from which to chart your course. You need only remember that there are four components to your successful future.

Knowledge is the first component. Whether you learn the basic tools of pharmacy in the classroom, at the job site, or from books on your own, you have the key to opening a door of exciting challenges.

Your *Experience* will be your second component. Real world experience provides the ultimate practical learning environment. Some call it "street-savvy"; this will enable you to deal with real people in a real way. As you become an effective participant in health-care delivery, you will serve well both the patient individually and the society as a whole.

The third component is *Self-pacing*. We never dispense guesswork. Pace yourself until you understand what must be understood. Proceed only when you feel comfortable. Your grasp of the knowledge will assure your success on the certification exam, in the workplace, and within yourself. The extra time is a small price to invest for a fulfilling future.

Finally, there is the component of *Self-presentation*. This is an attitude that enables you to walk proudly among other professionals. Think professionally, act professionally, speak professionally, and present yourself professionally.

Good luck in your career.

Marvin M. Stoogenke, R.Ph.

Acknowledgments

I would like to express my appreciation and thanks to my family for their continuing support of my writing activities. Thanks go to my sons Scott, Jason, and Saul, who never cease to lend an ear and a word. Special thanks go to my wife, Judy, as well as Saul, whose seemingly tireless typing of the manuscript assured its timeliness.

Judy, your perseverance and energy keep me going regardless of my thoughts on the matter. You give me purpose and you are my purpose. Thank you. I love you. MWA

Additionally, I extend my gratitude to the Pharmacy Technician Certification Board visionaries who were able to see the role pharmacy technicians would play in an evolutionary health-care delivery system, and who have pioneered to define the role and importance qualified pharmacy technicians have in the health of society.

Marvin M. Stoogenke, R.Ph.

Introduction

SUCCESS ACROSS THE BOARDS: THE PRENTICE HALL HEALTH REVIEW SERIES

Prentice Hall is pleased to present *Success Across the Boards,* our new review series. These authoritative texts give you expert help in preparing for certifying examinations. Each title in the series comes with its own technology package, including a CD-ROM and a Companion Website. You will find that this powerful combination of text and media provides you with expert help and guidance for achieving success across the boards. This outline review for the dental assistant provides help for preparing for the Certified Dental Assistant Examinations in General Chairside, Infection Control, Radiation Health and Safety, Certified Orthodontic Assistant, and Certified Dental Practice Management Administrator.

COMPONENTS OF THE SERIES

The series is made up of one book and CD combination.

About the Book: *Question and Answer Review for the Pharmacy Technician* by Marvin Stoogenke and Peter Le

- *Study Questions:* The book has been designed to help the student prepare for the written certification exam. There are over 1,000 multiple choice questions, which are organized by the all the topics covered on the exam and follow the exam format. Working through these questions will help you assess your strengths and weaknesses in each topic of study. Correct answers and comprehensive rationales are included.

About the CD-ROM

A CD-ROM is included in the back of this book. The CD-ROM is intended as a practice exam. Correct answers and comprehensive rationales and references follow all questions. You will receive immediate feedback to identify your strengths and weaknesses in each topic covered.

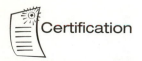

Certification

The Pharmacy Technician Certification Board (PTCB) administers the certification exam nationally. Once you are certified, you are required to obtain 20 hours of continuing education every 2 years in order to maintain your certification as being active. To obtain more information about the exam and the career of a pharmacy technician, visit the following website: *http://www.ptcb.org/* or you may contact the PTCB through the following address and phone number:

Pharmacy Technician Certification Board
2215 Constitution Avenue, NW
Washington, DC 20037-2985
Phone: (202) 429-7576
Fax: (202) 429-7596

If at all possible, the best way would be to visit the website. The website gives in-depth information about the exam, exam schedule, practice exam, and will allow you to register online for the upcoming exams, information about recertification, and it is a fast and convenient way to get information you may need or want. Even though there is not a federal law mandating pharmacy technicians to be certified, most institutions, if not states, would prefer or even require technicians to be certified in order to work in a pharmacy.

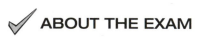

ABOUT THE EXAM

The Pharmacy Technician Certification Exam is given three times a year and it is administered nationally. The exam was started in 1995 and to date over 131,000 technicians have been certified nationally. The cost for an exam is $120. Check the website or contact the certification board for the exam schedule, since the dates do change on a yearly basis.

As for the exam itself, it covers three broad functional areas:

    I. Assisting the Pharmacist in Serving Patients—64% of Examination

   II. Maintaining Medication and Inventory Control Systems—25% of Examination

 III. Participating in the Administration and Management of Pharmacy Practice—11% of Examination

Once again, please refer to the website for more information about the exam.

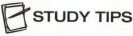

STUDY TIPS

Review Materials

Choose review materials that contain the information you need to study. Save time by making sure you aren't studying anything you don't need to. Before the exam, the best study preparation would be to use this Question & Answer Review to identify your strengths and weaknesses. The references at the end of each rationale will direct you to additional resources for more in-depth study.

Set a Study Schedule

Use your time-management skills to set a schedule that will help you feel as prepared as you can be. Consider all the relevant factors—the materials you need to study, how many months, weeks, or days until the test date, and how much time you can study each day. If you establish your schedule ahead of time and write it in your date book, you will be much more likely to follow it.

Take Practice Tests

Practice as much as possible, using the questions in this book, on the accompanying CD, and the Web. These questions were designed to follow the format of questions that appear on the exam you will take, so the more you practice with these questions, the better prepared you will be on test day.

The printed practice test in the back of the book and the practice tests on the CD will give you a chance to experience the exam before you actually have to take it and will also let you know how you're doing and where you need to do better. For best results, we recommend you take a practice test 2 to 3 weeks before you are scheduled to take the actual exam. Spend the next weeks targeting those areas in which you performed poorly by reviewing questions in those areas.

Practice under test-like conditions—in a quiet room, with no books or notes to help you, and with a clock telling you when to quit. Try to come as close as you can to duplicating the actual test situation.

TAKING THE EXAMINATION

Prepare Physically

When taking the exam, you need to work efficiently under time pressure. If your body is tired or under stress, you might not think as clearly or perform as well as you usually do. If you can, avoid staying up all night. Get some sleep so you wake up rested and alert.

Eating right is also important. The best advice is to eat a light, well-balanced meal before a test. When time is short, grab a quick-energy snack such as a banana, orange juice, or a granola bar.

The Examination Site

The examination site must be located prior to the required examination time. One suggestion is to find the site and parking facilities the day before the test. Parking fee information should be obtained so sufficient money can be taken along on the examination day.

Allow plenty of time for travel to the site in case of unexpected mishaps such as traffic snarls. During travel, think positive thoughts (e.g., "My preparation for the exam was thorough, so I'll be able to answer the questions easily"). Maintain a confident attitude to prevent unnecessary stress.

Materials

Be sure to take all required identification materials, registration forms, and any other items required by the testing organization or center. Read information and instructions supplied by the testing organizations thoroughly to be sure you have all necessary materials before the day of the exam.

Read Test Directions

Read the examination directions thoroughly! Because some board examinations have different test sections with different question formats, it is important to be aware of changes in directions. Read each set of directions completely before starting a new section of questions.

Machine-scored tests require you use a special pencil to fill in a small box on a computerized answer sheet. Use the right pencil (usually a number 2), and mark your answers in the correct space. Neatness counts on these tests, because the computer can misread stray pencil marks or partially erased answers. Periodically check the answer number against the question number to make sure they match. One question skipped can cause every answer following it to be marked incorrect.

Selecting the Right Answer

Keep in mind only one answer is correct. First read the stem of the question with *each* possible choice provided and eliminate choices that are obviously incorrect. Be cautious about choosing the first answer that *might* be correct; all possibilities should be considered before the final choice is made; the best answer should be selected.

If a question is complicated, try to break it down into small sections that are easy to understand. Pay special attention to qualifiers such as *only, except,* etc. For example, negative words in a question can confuse your understanding of what the question asks ("Which of the following is *not. . .*").

Intelligent Guessing

If you don't know the answer, eliminate those answers that you know or suspect are wrong. Your goal is to narrow down your choices. Here are some questions to ask yourself:

- Is the choice accurate in its own terms? If there's an error in the choice, for example, a term that is incorrectly defined—the answer is wrong.
- Is the choice relevant? An answer may be accurate, but it may not relate to the essence of the question.
- Are there any distractors, such as *always, never, all, none,* or *every?* Qualifiers make it easy to find an exception that makes a choice incorrect.

Mark answers you aren't sure of, and go back to them at the end of the test. Ask yourself whether you would make the same guesses again. Chances are you will leave your answers alone, but you may notice something that will make you change your mind—a qualifier that affects meaning or a remembered fact that will enable you to answer the question without guessing.

Watch the Clock

Keep track of how much time is left and how you are progressing. Wear a watch or bring a small clock with you to the test room. A wall clock may be broken, or there may be no clock at all.

Some students are so concerned about time, they rush through the exam and have time left over. In such situations, it's easy to leave early. The best approach, however, is to take your time. Stay until the end so that you can check your answers.

KEYS TO SUCCESS ACROSS THE BOARDS

- Study, Review, and Practice
- Keep a positive, confident attitude
- Follow all directions on the examination
- Do your best

Good luck!

You are encouraged to visit http://www.prenhall.com/success *for additional tips on studying, test-taking, and other keys to success. At this stage of your education and career you will find these tips helpful.*

Some of the study and test-taking tips were adapted from Keys to Effective Learning, *Second Edition by Carol Carter, Joyce Bishop, and Sarah Lyman Kravits.*

Stoogenke Reviewers

Davis M. Baker, B.S. Pharm., MBA, JD
Professor and Chair
Pharmacy Science and Technology Department
Holyoke Community College
Holyoke, Massachusetts

Anirwddh Hathi
Associate Professor
Pharmacy Technology
Texas State Technical College–Waco
Texas, Waco

Barbara Lacher BS, RphTech, CPhT
Associate Professor and Assistant Program Director
Pharmacy Technology
North Dakota State College of Science
Wahpeton, North Dakota

Ramona Mulleins, BSN
Instructor
Pharmacy Technology
Columbus Technical College
Columbus, Georgia

Darlene Redd, CPhT
Instructor
Pharmacy Technician Program
Tennessee Technology Center at Jackson
Jackson, Tennessee

Marsha M. Sanders, BS, RPh
Pharmacy Technology Director
Jones County Junior College
Ellisville, Missouri

Lyndi C. Shadbolt, MS, BSN, RN
Assistant Professor
Pharmacy Technology Program Coordinator
Amarillo College
Amarillo, Texas

Mark Williams, BS, CPhT
Coordinator
Pharmacy Technology Program
Mercy College of Northwest Ohio
Toledo, Ohio

1 Assisting the Pharmacist in Serving Patient Medications

chapter objectives

Students will demonstrate knowledge of:

➤ The brand and generic names of commonly prescribed medications

➤ The primary uses of commonly prescribed medications

➤ The usual dosing of commonly prescribed medications

➤ The common side effects of commonly prescribed medications

➤ The notable interactions of commonly prescribed medications

➤ The important special information relevant to commonly prescribed medications

➤ The classifications and groupings of commonly prescribed medications

DIRECTIONS Each of the questions or incomplete statements below is followed by suggested answers or completions. Select the **one answer** that is best in each case.

1. Ergotamine is to CAFERGOT as sucralfate is to _____?
   A. BANTHINE
   B. QUARZAN
   C. CARAFATE
   D. ROBINAL

2. Which of the following answers best describes a primary indicated use for enalapril?
   A. atherosclerosis
   B. arrhythmia
   C. hypertension
   D. bradycardia

3. What is the brand name for ketorolac?
   A. TORADOL
   B. TOBREX
   C. TOFRANIL
   D. KYTRIL

4. Which of the following is the generic name for PREMARIN?
   A. tamoxifen
   B. norethindrone
   C. ethinyl estradiol
   D. conjugated estrogens

5. ORTHO-NOVUM is to NORINYL as diltiazem is to _____?
   A. phenobarbital
   B. verapamil
   C. hydantoin
   D. ranitidine

6. Which of the following answers best describes the most common indication for fluoxetine?
   A. bipolar affective disorders (BAD)
   B. seasonal affective disorders (SAD)
   C. hypertension
   D. major depression

7. Which is the generic name for HUMULIN?
   A. insulin
   B. glipizide
   C. glyburide
   D. chlorpropamide

8. How would you classify or group sertraline?
   A. NSAID
   B. HMG-CoA
   C. TCA
   D. SSRI

9. Which is a trade name for penicillin VK?
   A. VERELAN
   B. PENTIDS
   C. V-CILLIN K
   D. VISKEN

10. How would you classify or group levothyroxine?
    A. hypoglycemic agent
    B. thyroid hormone
    C. corticosteroid
    D. contraceptive agent

11. Which of the following is the generic name for COUMADIN?
    A. warfarin
    B. hydrocortisone
    C. triamcinolone
    D. cortisone

12. Which of the following is a side effect reported with sertraline?
    A. loss of muscle coordination
    B. chest pain
    C. dry mouth
    D. rash

13. Which of the following is the trade name for loratidine?
    A. ATARAX
    B. CLARITIN
    C. ALLEGRA
    D. BENADRYL

14. Which of the following answers best describes the usual oral dosage for loratidine?
    A. 10 mg daily
    B. 10 mg BID
    C. 20 mg daily
    D. titrate dose as needed

15. Which is an appropriate auxiliary label to use with nabumetone?
    A. Avoid alcohol.
    B. Avoid aspirin.
    C. Take with food or milk.
    D. All of the above

16. Which of the following answers best describes the primary indicated use for ethinyl estradiol/levonorgestrel?
    A. inactive thyroid
    B. hypoglycemia
    C. prostatic cancer
    D. prevention of pregnancy

17. How would you classify or group penicillin VK?
    A. antifungal
    B. anti-infective
    C. antiprotozoal
    D. antiulcer

18. Which is an appropriate auxiliary label to use with verapamil (sustained release form)?
    A. Take with food.
    B. Do not crush.
    C. Store in glass.
    D. A and B

19. Which of the following is the generic name for PRILOSEC?
    A. pantoprazole
    B. lansoprazole
    C. omeprezole
    D. rabeprazole

20. Which of the following best describes a unique characteristic for colchicine?
    A. causes localized rash
    B. overdose causes hair loss
    C. causes heartburn
    D. impairs the absorption of vitamin B_{12}

21. Is nizatidine available as an OTC?
    A. yes
    B. no
    C. pending
    D. under FDA review

22. What information should you give the patient taking simvastatin?
    A. Use in conjunction with dietary therapy.
    B. Double missed doses.
    C. Report muscle pain, fever, weakness.
    D. A and C

23. What is the generic name for ADALAT?
    A. nisoldipine
    B. nizatidine
    C. acebutolol
    D. nifedipine

24. Which of the following drugs is a selective serotonin reuptake inhibitor (SSRI)?
    A. diazepam
    B. chlorpromazine
    C. fluoxetine
    D. haloperidol

25. Which of the following answers best describes the primary indicated use of verapamil?
    A. edema
    B. angina, hypertension
    C. TIA
    D. MI, CHF

26. Which is a trade name for triamterene/hydrochlorothiazide?
    A. MAXZIDE
    B. DIUPRES
    C. DYAZIDE
    D. A and C

27. Clonidine is to _____ as quinidine is to QUINORA.
    A. TENEX
    B. CATAPRES
    C. ALDOMET
    D. WYTENSIN

28. Coadministration of simvastatin and which of the following may produce an unwanted result?
    A. herbal medications
    B. gemfibrozil
    C. loperamide
    D. diphenoxylate

29. Which of the following answers best describes the primary indications for ranitidine?
    A. treat angina, hypertension
    B. treat hypercholesterolemia

C. treat depression, obsessive–compulsive disorder
D. treat duodenal ulcer, gastroesophageal reflux, and gastric hypersecretory conditions

30. Which of the following is the generic name for LASIX?
    A. bumetanide
    B. amiloride
    C. spironolactone
    D. furosemide

31. Which of the following answers best describes the primary indicated use for ethinyl estradiol/norethindrone?
    A. prevention of pregnancy
    B. supplement to breast cancer treatment
    C. prostatic carinoma
    D. inactive thyroid

32. Which best describes the usual adult dose for clonazepam?
    A. up to 5 cc/day
    B. not to exceed 10 units/d
    C. 1.5 mg/day in three divided doses
    D. maximum 20 mg/day

33. What is the brand name for pravastatin?
    A. PROCARDIA
    B. PRECOSE
    C. PRONESTYL
    D. PRAVACHOL

34. Which of the following is the generic name for PLAQUENIL?
    A. hydroxocobalamin
    B. plicamycin
    C. hydroxyprogesterone
    D. hydroxychloroquine

35. What is the usual adult dose of PLAVIX?
    A. 150 mg/day

B. 300 mg/day

C. 75 mg/day

D. 1 mg/kg q12h

36. Which of the following is a common side effect reported with clonazepam?

A. drowsiness

B. tachycardia

C. bradycardia

D. rash

37. Which of the following is the generic name for PROZAC?

A. fluconazole

B. fluoxetine

C. fluphenazine

D. flurazepam

38. Which of the following is the generic name for TAXOL?

A. pamidronate

B. paclitaxel

C. pancrelipase

D. tamoxifen

39. Which of the following answers best describes a unique association with nifedipine?

A. Take medication with plenty of fluid.

B. Do not chew or break sustained-release dosage form.

C. Store in glass.

D. Limit time spent in sunlight.

40. Coadministration of glipizide and which of the following may produce an unwanted result?

A. TCN

B. PCN

C. NSAIDs

D. DPH

41. Which of the following is the trade name for glipizide?

A. DIABETA

B. GLUCOTROL

C. ORINASE

D. TOLINASE

42. Which of the following is a side effect reported with penicillin VK?

A. bruising

B. thirst

C. diarrhea

D. muscle cramps

43. How would you classify or group simvastatin?

A. antiemetic agent

B. antihyperlipidemic agent

C. antidiarrheal agent

D. anti-inflammatory agent

44. Using the key phrase "gastric acid secretion" as the basis for your decision, which of the following does not belong?

A. diphenhydramine

B. omeprazole

C. nizatidine

D. cimetidine

45. Which of the following is the generic name for DIFLUCAN?

A. ketoconazole

B. fluconazole

C. itraconazole

D. miconazole

46. "Azepam" in the name of a drug best describes which of the following types of drugs?

A. beta lactams

B. benzodiazepines

C. steroids

D. tricylic antidepressants

47. Which of the following answers best describes the most common indication(s) for omeprazole?
    A. gastroenteritis
    B. angina, hypertension
    C. Crohn's disease
    D. erosive esophagitis and gastroesophageal reflux disease

48. Which of the following answers best describes the primary indicated use for sertraline?
    A. cardiovascular disease
    B. major depression
    C. peptic ulcer disease
    D. chronic obstructive pulmonary disease

49. Which of the following answers best describes the usual dosage for paclitaxel?
    A. 500 mg/kg every 8 hours
    B. 250 mg every 4 hours
    C. 135–175 mg/m^2 over 3 hours every 3 weeks
    D. 1 gm bolus

50. Which is an appropriate auxiliary label to use with penicillin VK?
    A. Take with orange juice.
    B. Finish all this medication unless otherwise directed by prescriber.
    C. May cause drowsiness.
    D. May cause discoloration of urine or feces.

51. Which of the following is a side effect reported with hydroxychloroquine?
    A. digital numbness
    B. joint pains
    C. gastrointestinal disturbance
    D. sweats

52. Which is an appropriate auxiliary label to use with methotrexate?

    A. Take on an empty stomach.
    B. Take with food.
    C. Do not crush.
    D. Avoid smoking while taking this medication.

53. Which of the following is a side effect reported with simvastatin?
    A. abdominal cramps
    B. constipation
    C. headache
    D. all of the above

54. Amoxicillin may diminish the action of which group of drugs?
    A. antidepressants
    B. steroids
    C. oral contraceptives
    D. antihistamines

55. Which of the following is the generic name for ANAPROX?
    A. nalaxone
    B. amrinone
    C. naproxen
    D. nandrolone

56. What information should you give the patient taking ethinyl estradiol/levonorgestrel?
    A. Reduce dietary fiber while taking this medication.
    B. Discontinue if you are pregnant or intend to become pregnant.
    C. Double missed doses.
    D. Skip a dose if experiencing vision disturbance.

57. What medication would you use for urinary tract pain/discomfort?
    A. colchicine
    B. phenazopyridine
    C. urease
    D. ibuprofen

58. Using the key word "lipids" as the basis for your decision, which of the following does not belong?
    A. lovastatin
    B. gemfibrozil
    C. nicotinic acid
    D. nystatin

59. Which is an appropriate auxiliary label to use with warfarin?
    A. May cause discoloration of the urine or feces.
    B. Do not take dairy products while taking this medication.
    C. Avoid prolonged exposure to sunlight.
    D. Take with food or milk.

60. What is the trade name for lisinopril?
    A. ZESTRIL
    B. DIURIL
    C. PRINVIL
    D. A and C

61. What is the generic name for the drug CECLOR?
    A. cephalexin
    B. cephradine
    C. cefuroxime
    D. cefaclor

62. Which of the following is the trade name for cyclophosphamide?
    A. CYLERT
    B. CYTOXAN
    C. CYTADREN
    D. CYTOGAM

63. Which of the following is the generic name for PEPCID?
    A. ranitidine
    B. cimetidine
    C. famotidine
    D. nizatidine

64. What information should you give the patient or caregiver about taking ciprofloxacin?
    A. May cause drowsiness.
    B. Do not crush tablets.
    C. May be habit-forming.
    D. Do not take with dairy products.

65. Coadministration of penicillin VK and which of the following may produce an unwanted result?
    A. atenolol
    B. carisoprodol
    C. tetracycline
    D. sertraline

66. Cimetidine is contraindicated in patients treated with which of the following?
    A. theophylline
    B. warfarin
    C. zolpidem
    D. A and B

67. Which of the following answers best describes the most common indication(s) for NORVASC?
    A. hypertension
    B. hypercholesterolemia
    C. hypercalcemia
    D. hypernatremia

68. Which of the following answers best describes the usual adult oral dosage for phenytoin?
    A. maintenance dose: one capsule TID or QID
    B. maximum dose: two capsules TID
    C. once-a-day dose: 300 mg of the extended release form
    D. all of the above

69. Which of the following is a common side effect reported with diclofenac use?
    A. headache
    B. gastrointestinal disturbance
    C. lightheadedness
    D. loss of hair

70. Which of the following is the generic name for TRIPHASIL 28?
    A. ethinyl estradiol
    B. ethinyl estradiol/levonorgestrel
    C. conjugated estrogens
    D. ethinyl estradiol/norethindrone

71. Coadministration of warfarin and which of the following may result in a potentially serious or even life-threatening drug interaction?
    A. barbiturates
    B. H2 antagonists
    C. sulfa antibiotics
    D. all of the above

72. What should you ask a patient who is about to receive BACTRIM?
    A. Have you taken this medication before?
    B. Do you know why you are taking BACTRIM?
    C. Are you allergic to sulfa-drugs?
    D. All of the above

73. Using the key phrase "gram positive" as the basis for your decision, which of the following does not belong?
    A. cephalosporins
    B. penicillins
    C. erythromycin
    D. metronidazole

74. Coadministration of furosemide and which of the following may produce an unwanted result?
    A. steroids

B. analgesics
C. hypoglycemic agents
D. histamine H2 antagonists

75. Using the key phrase "seasonal allergy" as the basis for your decision, which of the following does not belong?
    A. diphenhydramine
    B. phenytoin
    C. loratidine
    D. fexofenidine

76. Which of the following is the trade name for loratidine?
    A. CLAFORAN
    B. CLEOCIN
    C. LOPID
    D. CLARITIN

77. Which of the following is the generic name for VASOTEC?
    A. enalapril
    B. verapamil
    C. lisinopril
    D. amlodipine

78. Which of the following is the trade name for prazosin?
    A. MINOCIN
    B. PRILOSEC
    C. MINIPRESS
    D. MONOPRIL

79. Which of the following answers best describes the primary indicated use for insulin?
    A. diabetes insipidus
    B. lipoatrophic diabetes
    C. insulin-dependent diabetes mellitus
    D. noninsulin-dependent diabetes mellitus

80. What is the brand name for amiodarone?
    A. ADENOCARD

B. CORDARONE

C. NORVASC

D. CORGARD

81. Which of the following is the generic name for RELAFEN?
    A. ranitidine
    B. nadolol
    C. rifampin
    D. nabumetone

82. Which of the following drug classes or groups is represented by oxaprozin?
    A. analgesics (opiate)
    B. anti-inflammatory agents (NSAID)
    C. psychotherapeutic agents (tranquilizer)
    D. cardiovascular agents (ACE inhibitor)

83. Which of the following drug classes or groups is represented by cefepime?
    A. first-generation cephalosporin
    B. second-generation cephalosporin
    C. third-generation cephalosporin
    D. fourth-generation cephalosporin

84. Which best describes the usual adult dose for colchicine?
    A. 8 mg BID
    B. maximum of 8 mg per course of therapy
    C. 2 mg TID
    D. up to 4 mg per day separated by 3-day intervals

85. Which of the following is the generic name for ZOFRAN?
    A. zolpidem
    B. ofloxacin
    C. omeprazole
    D. ondansetron

86. Which of the following is a common side effect reported with drugs containing the ingredient oxycodone?
    A. hypotension

B. ototoxicity

C. drowsiness

D. insomnia

87. Which of the following is the generic name for DYAZIDE?
    A. triamterene
    B. chlorothiazide
    C. triamterene/hydrochlorothiazide
    D. bumetanide

88. Which is an appropriate auxiliary label to use with loratidine?
    A. Take with food.
    B. Finish all this medication unless otherwise directed by prescriber.
    C. May cause discoloration of urine or feces.
    D. Take on an empty stomach.

89. Ciprofloxacin works best when avoiding which of the following?
    A. antacids containing aluminum, magnesium, or calcium
    B. products containing zinc or iron
    C. caffeine
    D. all of the above

90. How would you classify or group eptifibatide?
    A. analgesic
    B. antiplatelet
    C. diuretic
    D. hormone

91. Using the key word "hyperglycemic" as the basis for your decision, which of the following does not belong?
    A. thirst
    B. visual disturbance
    C. excessive urination
    D. none of the above

92. What is the trade name for hydroxychloro-
    quine?
    A. HYDREA
    B. PLACIDYL
    C. PLAQUENIL
    D. PLENDIL

93. Which of the following is the generic name
    for VOLTAREN?
    A. dicloxacillin
    B. dicyclomine
    C. verapamil
    D. diclofenac

94. How would you classify or group penicil-
    lamine?
    A. antibiotic
    B. antiviral
    C. antifungal agent
    D. chelating agent

95. Which of the following answers best de-
    scribes the primary indicated use for ketoro-
    lac?
    A. cardiac arrhythmia
    B. indigestion
    C. GERD
    D. short-term pain management

96. What is the generic name for COREG?
    A. atenolol
    B. esmolol
    C. carvedilol
    D. carteolol

97. Which of the following best describes the
    primary indicated use for MAXALT?
    A. migraine heaches
    B. infections
    C. hyperglycemia
    D. insomnia

98. Which of the following drug classes or
    groups is represented by medroxyproges-
    terone?
    A. progestogens
    B. adrenal corticosteroids
    C. anabolic steroids
    D. estrogens

99. What is the generic name for BIAXIN?
    A. erythromycin
    B. clarithromycin
    C. streptomycin
    D. vancomycin

100. Which of the following answers best de-
     scribes the most common indication for
     AVAPRO?
     A. hyperglycemia
     B. depression
     C. erectile dysfunction
     D. hypertension

101. What is the primary indication for
     pramipexole?
     A. depression
     B. Alzheimer's disease
     C. hypersecretory disease of GI tract
     D. Parkinson's disease

102. What is the dose for ZAROXOLYN when
     used for hypertension?
     A. 2.5–5 mg
     B. 10 mg
     C. 0.5 mg/kg
     D. 1.5 mg/kg

103. What information should you emphasize to
     the patient taking glyburide?
     A. the importance of good foot care
     B. the importance of immediate care for
        cuts and bruises

C. the importance of not skipping meals

D. all of the above

104. What is/are the indication(s) for FOS-AMAX?

A. osteoporosis

B. Paget's disease

C. nausea and vomiting

D. A and B

105. Which of the following is a side effect reported with CLARITIN?

A. glossitis

B. rapid heart rate

C. memory loss

D. dry mouth

106. What is the trade or brand name for the generic drug captopril?

A. VASOTEC

B. MONOPRIL

C. LOTENSIN

D. CAPOTEN

107. All of the following drugs are available as transdermal patches except

A. nitroglycerin

B. dopamine

C. nicotine

D. clonidine

108. Using the key word "insulin" as the basis for your decision, which of the following does not belong?

A. glyburide

B. glipizide

C. furosemide

D. tolazamide

109. Which answer best describes the usual adult dose for paroxetine?

A. 50 mg qhs

B. up to 50 mcg per day

C. 25 mcg BID

D. maximum 50 mg per day

110. Which of the following is the trade name for furosemide?

A. LASIX

B. LANOXIN

C. LEVADOPA

D. FORTAZ

111. What information should you give the patient taking triamterene/hydrochlorothiazide?

A. Supplement your diet with one banana per day.

B. Take medication early enough during the day to prevent nocturia.

C. Double your vitamin intake per day.

D. Double up on missed doses.

112. Which of the following is the generic name for KLONOPIN?

A. clonazepam

B. clorazepate

C. clonidine

D. clozapine

113. How would you classify or group hydroxychloroquine?

A. antimalarial agent

B. cardiovascular agent

C. musculoskeletal agent

D. psychotherapeutic agent

114. What is the trade or brand name for the generic drug paclitaxel?

A. PAXIL

B. TAXOL

C. TALWIN

D. PARLODEL

115. What is the generic name for the drug GLUCOPHAGE?
   A. glyburide
   B. metformin
   C. glipizide
   D. methylergonovine

116. Which drug category or class does ZANAFLEX belong to?
   A. antibiotic
   B. antihypertensive
   C. muscle relaxant
   D. diuretic

117. What is the trade or brand name for the generic drug medroxyprogesterone?
   A. OGEN
   B. MICRONOR
   C. PROVERA
   D. OVRETTE

118. Using the word "cholesterol," which of the following does not belong with the others?
   A. pravastatin
   B. cholestyramine
   C. celecoxib
   D. niacin

119. What information should you give the patient taking diclofenac?
   A. Do not crush tablets.
   B. Take with food or milk.
   C. Report signs of blood in the stools.
   D. All of the above

120. Which answer best describes the usual adult dose for ibuprofen?
   A. 800 mg daily
   B. two tablets qid
   C. 400 mg qhs
   D. maximum 3.2 gm per day

121. What is the generic name for the drug NEO-SYNEPHRINE?
   A. dopamine
   B. pseudoephedrine
   C. norepinephrine
   D. phenylephrine

122. The drug allopurinol is to gout as _____ is to smoking cessation treatment.
   A. phenobarbital
   B. bupropion
   C. betaxolol
   D. promethazine

123. Which is an appropriate auxiliary label to use with medroxyprogesterone?
   A. Do not crush.
   B. Avoid prolonged exposure to sunlight while taking this medication.
   C. Take on an empty stomach.
   D. May cause drowsiness.

124. Using the word "glaucoma," which of the following does not belong with the others?
   A. naphazoline
   B. timolol
   C. pilocarpine
   D. carbachol

125. What is the brand name for propoxyphene napsylate/acetaminophen?
   A. DARVOCET-N
   B. DARVON-N
   C. DARVON COMPOUND
   D. DECADRON

126. Which of the following would be considered a non-narcotic analgesic?
   A. VICODIN
   B. LORTAB
   C. ULTRAM
   D. PERCOCET

127. Which of the following is used to "counter-attack" the effects of COUMADIN?
    A. heparin
    B. phytonadione
    C. warfarin
    D. thiamine

128. How would you classify or group ZYPREXA?
    A. NSAID
    B. laxative
    C. antipsychotic
    D. antispasmotic

129. Which of the following answers best describes a unique association with glipizide?
    A. increased risk of cardiovascular mortality
    B. increased risk of impotence
    C. increased risk of ototoxicity
    D. increased risk of irreversible visual dysfunction

130. Which of the following asthma medications must be taken regularly and is not intended for acute exacerbations?
    A. PROVENTIL
    B. VENTOLIN
    C. BRICANYL
    D. SINGULAIR

131. Which of the following is the trade name for amphotericin B?
    A. NIZORAL
    B. SPORANOX
    C. LOTRIMIN
    D. ABELCET

132. Which of the following is the generic name for SEROQUEL?
    A. quetiapine
    B. orphenadrine
    C. olanzapine
    D. citalopram

133. What is the generic name for the drug CIPRO?
    A. ofloxacin
    B. ciprofloxacin
    C. lomefloxacin
    D. norfloxacin

134. What warning label should be on bottles of PREMARIN?
    A. May cause drowsiness.
    B. Avoid prolonged exposure to sunlight.
    C. Take with food.
    D. Refrigerate.

135. Which of the following drugs does not have to be refrigerated?
    A. insulin
    B. fosphenytoin
    C. doxycycline
    D. sandostatin

136. Which of the following drugs does not have an oral dosage form?
    A. vancomycin
    B. cephalexin
    C. metoclopramide
    D. cefazolin

137. BENADRYL is to BENTYL as antihistamine is to _____?
    A. antidepressant
    B. antibiotic
    C. antispasmodic
    D. antihypertensive

138. Which of the following answers best describes the most common indication(s) for diltiazem?
    A. edema
    B. angina, hypertension
    C. congestive heart failure, MI
    D. atherosclerosis

139. Which of the following answers best describes the usual oral dosage for ciprofloxacin?
    A. Dose and frequency depend on the type and severity of the infection.
    B. All doses have a schedule of q12h.
    C. Daily doses range from 500–1500 mg.
    D. All of the above

140. Which of the following is a common side effect reported with cyclophosphamide use?
    A. headache
    B. lightheadedness
    C. dizziness
    D. hair loss

141. Calcium channel blockers are contraindicated in patients treated with which of the following?
    A. quinine medications
    B. quinapril
    C. quinidine products
    D. quinestrol

142. Which of the following drugs is contraindicated in pregnancy?
    A. CYTOTEC
    B. PITOCIN
    C. MAGNESIUM SALTS
    D. METHERGINE

143. Which of the following is available in IV and oral dosage forms?
    A. PRILOSEC
    B. PROTONIX
    C. ACIPHEX
    D. NEXIUM

144. Which of the following answers best describes the primary indicated use for naproxen?
    A. Rheumatoid arthritis (RA)
    B. dysmenorrhea

C. inflammatory disease
D. all of the above

145. All of the following are ingredients in FIORICET except
    A. acetaminophen
    B. aspirin
    C. butalbital
    D. caffeine

146. What is the brand name for ibuprofen?
    A. ORUDIS
    B. RELAFEN
    C. MOTRIN
    D. DAYPRO

147. What do phenelzine and tranylcypromine have in common?
    A. MAO inhibitors
    B. SSR inhibitors
    C. NSAIDs
    D. TCAs

148. What information should you give the patient taking verapamil?
    A. Limit caffeine intake.
    B. Maintain a low-sodium diet.
    C. Use available techniques to deal with stress.
    D. All of the above

149. Using the key term "volume expander" as the basis for your answer, which of the following does not belong?
    A. ALBUMINAR
    B. HESPAN
    C. ALDACTONE
    D. PLASMANATE

150. The usual dose for ARICEPT for adults is
    A. 50 mg qhs
    B. 5 mg tid

C. 10 mg bid prn

D. 5–10 mg qhs

151. Elavil is to amitriptyline as _____ is to MELLARIL.

A. theophylline

B. thioridazine

C. thiothixene

D. thiopental

152. What is the usual adult oral dose for diltiazem?

A. capsules, up to 500 mg per day

B. tablets, up to 600 mg per day

C. tablets or capsules, 180 mg per day

D. Optimum maintenance dose should not exceed 360 mg/day

153. Beta blockers are contraindicated in patients treated with which of the following?

A. clonidine

B. cladribine

C. clemastine

D. none of the above

154. What is the brand name of enoxaparin?

A. NORMIFLO

B. LOVENOX

C. FRAGMIN

D. WARFARIN

155. Which of the following antibiotics is used for urinary tract infections?

A. MACRODANTIN

B. VANCOCIN

C. ANCEF

D. FLAGYL

156. Which teratogenic drug is approved for limited use in patients with leprosy?

A. linezolid

B. thalidomide

C. rifampin

D. amikacin

157. Which is a trade name for verapamil?

A. PROCARDIA

B. NIMOTOP

C. VERELAN

D. none of the above

158. INDOCIN is to indomethacin as _____ is to MINOCIN.

A. minocycline

B. minoxidil

C. miconazole

D. metronidazole

159. What do fluoxetine, sertraline, and paroxetine have in common?

A. MAO inhibitors

B. ACE inhibitors

C. SSR inhibitors

D. proton pump inhibitors

160. What information should you give the patient taking ketorolac?

A. Watch for and report signs of adverse gastrointestinal events.

B. Limit use of oral form to 5 days.

C. Double dose for enhanced pain relief.

D. Take aspirin to boost the effectiveness.

161. Which of the following contains an antihistamine and a decongestant only?

A. ENTEX

B. HUMIBID DM

C. ALLEGRA-D

D. PHENERGAN VC WITH CODEINE

162. Which of the following is the trade name for filgrastim?

A. EPOGEN

B. PROCRIT

C. NEUMEGA

D. NEUPOGEN

163. Using the key phrase "thyroid gland" as the basis for your decision, which of the following does not belong?
    A. levothyroxine
    B. iodine
    C. idoxuridine
    D. goiter

164. Which of the following is the generic name for MEVACOR?
    A. lovastatin
    B. pravastatin
    C. simvastatin
    D. gemfibrozil

165. ACE inhibitors are contraindicated in patients treated with which of the following?
    A. prednisone
    B. potassium products
    C. potassium-sparing diuretics
    D. B and C

166. What is the generic name for PHOSLO?
    A. calcium gluconate
    B. calcium carbonate
    C. calcium chloride
    D. calcium acetate

167. Which of the following drug classes or groups is represented by captopril?
    A. cardiovasculars (ACE inhibitors)
    B. cardiovasculars (calcium channel blockers)
    C. cardiovasculars (vasodilators)
    D. respiratory agents (beta antagonists)

168. How would you classify or group verapamil?
    A. ACE inhibitor
    B. beta-adrenergic blocker
    C. inotropic agent
    D. calcium channel blocker

169. Which of the following answers best describes the primary indicated use for loratidine?
    A. angina
    B. hypercholesterolemia
    C. relieves symptoms of seasonal allergy
    D. edema

170. What is the usual starting dose for GLU-COPHAGE?
    A. 500 mg qd bid
    B. 1000 mg tid
    C. 250 mg qd
    D. 1000 mg q8h prn

171. What do itraconazole, fluconazole, and ketoconazole have in common?
    A. They are "azoles."
    B. They are antifungal agents.
    C. Coadministration with phenytoin is contraindicated.
    D. all of the above

172. Methylphenidate is used for what condition?
    A. cough/cold
    B. pain/inflammation
    C. attention deficit disorder
    D. gout

173. Which of the following answers best describes a unique association with diclofenac?
    A. As an NSAID, it has an unwanted impact on the gastric lining.
    B. As an antibiotic, it has an unwanted impact on destroying intestinal flora.
    C. As an antineoplastic, it has an unwanted impact on hair loss.
    D. As an antihistamine, it has an unwanted impact on drowsiness.

174. Thiazide diuretic is to ZAROXOLYN as _____ is to ZEBETA.

A. ACE inhibitor

B. calcium channel blocker

C. inotrope

D. beta-blocker

175. Which of the following is the generic name for MUCOMYST?

A. acetylcholine

B. acetylcysteine

C. acetazolamide

D. abciximab

176. The drug NEOSPORIN contains all of the following ingredients except

A. trimethoprin

B. neomycin

C. bacitracin

D. polymixin B

177. Digoxin is contraindicated in patients treated with which of the following?

A. dexamethasone

B. diphenoxylate

C. phenazopyridine

D. amiodarone

178. Using the key word "ulceration" as the basis for your decision, which of the following does not belong?

A. ibuprofen

B. naproxen

C. aspirin

D. loperamide

179. What is the brand name for acyclovir?

A. ZOCOR

B. ZOVIRAX

C. ZOLOFT

D. ZANTAC

180. Which of the following is a side effect reported with verapamil?

A. bulging eyes

B. lightheadedness

C. numbness

D. tremor

181. Which of the following drug classes or groups is represented by phenytoin?

A. antiseizure agents (dicarbamates)

B. antiseizure agents (hydantoins)

C. antiseizure agents (succinimides)

D. psychotherapeutic agents (antidepressants)

182. Which of the following answers best describes the most common indication for amoxicillin?

A. infection caused by susceptible strains of pathogens

B. obsessive–compulsive disorder

C. peptic ulcer, duodenal

D. major depression

183. How would you classify or group ondansetron?

A. antiemetic agent

B. antineoplastic agent

C. anti-inflammatory agent

D. psychotherapeutic agent

184. Which answer best describes the usual adult therapeutic oral dose for enalapril used for hypertension?

A. 10–40 mg/day

B. 20 mg BID

C. 20 mg TID

D. 2.5 mg qhs

185. What information should you give a patient taking warfarin?

A. Report black stools.

B. Use a soft toothbrush.

C. Protect the medication from light.

D. all of the above

186. Which of the following is a side effect reported with nifedipine?
   A. flushing
   B. hallucinations
   C. rash
   D. chills

187. SURFAK is to laxatives as _____ is to anticonvulsants
   A. NAPHCON-A
   B. NIMOTOP
   C. NEURONTIN
   D. NORPLANT

188. Potassium-wasting diuretics could be dangerous if used in patients treated with which of the following?
   A. TCAs
   B. NSAIDs
   C. proton pump inhibitors
   D. benzodiazepines

189. Which of the following drugs is NOT used for bladder spasms?
   A. CARDURA
   B. URISPAS
   C. LEVSIN
   D. ANASPAZ

190. Using the key word "edema" as the basis for your decision, which of the following does not belong?
   A. nandrolone
   B. furosemide
   C. spironolactone
   D. chlorothiazide

191. All of the following can be used for nausea and vomiting except
   A. ANTIVERT
   B. PHENERGAN
   C. SYMMETREL
   D. ZOFRAN

192. Which of the following drugs is not a brand name for lithium carbonate?
   A. ESKALITH
   B. THORAZINE
   C. LITHOBID
   D. LITHONATE

193. All of the following drugs are available as an OTC product except
   A. ibuprofen
   B. ranitidine
   C. ketoprofen
   D. etodolac

194. Potassium-sparing diuretics are contraindicated in patients treated with which of the following?
   A. ACE inhibitors
   B. TCAs
   C. potassium preparations
   D. A and C

195. Which of the following is the generic name for DIOVAN?
   A. losartan
   B. valsartan
   C. irbesartan
   D. candesartan

196. What action does cefprozil elicit?
   A. bacteriostatic
   B. bactericidal
   C. gene alteration
   D. pathogen replacement

197. Which answer best describes the usual adult dose for omeprazole?
   A. not to exceed 360 mg/day depending on condition
   B. maintain at 300 mcg/day for any condition
   C. 360 mcg BID for all conditions
   D. 300 mcg qhs for all conditions

198. What is the brand name for sertraline?
    A. ZOCOR
    B. ZANTAC
    C. SERZONE
    D. ZOLOFT

199. Which of the following is a common side effect reported with enalapril use?
    A. hallucinations
    B. bruising
    C. cough
    D. fever

200. NSAIDs are contraindicated in patients treated with which of the following?
    A. antiprotozoal agents
    B. antihistamine agents
    C. warfarin anticoagulants
    D. muscle relaxants

201. Which of the following drugs is indicated for treatment of diarrhea?
    A. ondansetron
    B. diphenhydramine
    C. loperamide
    D. guaifenesin

202. Clarithromycin should never be used with which of the following?
    A. nonsedating antihistamines
    B. calcium channel blockers
    C. protease inhibitors
    D. coenzyme A reductase inhibitors

203. Using the key phrase "serotonin reuptake inhibitor" as the basis for your decision, which of the following does not belong?
    A. sertraline
    B. fluoxetine
    C. desipramine
    D. paroxetine

204. How would you classify or group warfarin?
    A. antiarrhythmic agent
    B. anticoagulant agent
    C. antianginal agent
    D. antianxiety agent

205. Many oral antidiabetic drugs may be contraindicated in patients treated with which of the following?
    A. meperidine
    B. allopurinol
    C. phenylbutazone
    D. acetaminophen

206. TRICOR is to antihyperlipidemia as _____ is to antiseizures.
    A. CELEXA
    B. CEREBYX
    C. CELEBREX
    D. CELESTONE

207. Nitroglycerin patches are to qd as clondine patches are to _____.
    A. bid
    B. tid
    C. qweek
    D. q5d

208. SLOW-K is available in which of the following strengths?
    A. 10 meq
    B. 20 meq
    C. 6.7 meq
    D. 8 meq

209. Which of the following is the most potent drug?
    A. betamethasone
    B. hydrocortisone
    C. desonide
    D. mometasone

210. Which of the following answers best describes the primary indicated use for warfarin?
   A. tachycardia
   B. heart palpitations
   C. blood clots
   D. bradycardia

211. Theophylline-type asthma drugs are contraindicated in patients treated with which of the following?
   A. vitamin B_{12} supplements
   B. hyperosmotic laxatives
   C. antidiabetic agents
   D. quinolone antibiotics

212. For the drug HYZAAR 25/12.5, what ingredient does the 12.5 mg correlate to?
   A. losartan
   B. enalapril
   C. hydrochlorothiazide
   D. verapamil

213. Which is a brand name for verapamil?
   A. PLENDIL
   B. ISOPTIN
   C. DYNACIRC
   D. CARDENE

214. BRETHINE is to terbutaline as BRETHAIRE is to _____.
   A. isoetharine
   B. terbutaline
   C. epinephrine
   D. ephedrine

215. Which of the following is a common side effect reported with famotidine use?
   A. dizziness
   B. headache
   C. change in bowel movements
   D. all of the above

216. What is a common dose for LEVAQUIN in adults?
   A. 500 mg IV qd
   B. 500 mg po qd
   C. 500 mg po bid
   D. both A and B

217. ZOLOFT is to 50 mg a day as PROZAC is to _____.
   A. 50–100 mg bid
   B. 20 mg qd
   C. maximum of 500 mg a day
   D. 20 mg qid

218. Which is a side effect reported with warfarin use?
   A. blurred vision
   B. hair loss
   C. thirst
   D. tinnitus

219. Which is an appropriate strip label to use with paroxetine?
   A. May cause drowsiness.
   B. Do not crush or chew medication.
   C. Avoid alcohol.
   D. A and C

220. The antihypertensive drug minoxidil can also be found in what other product?
   A. ALDARA
   B. PROPECIA
   C. ROGAINE
   D. VIAGRA

221. Using the key phrase "fungal infection" as the basis for your decision, which of the following does not belong?
   A. fluconazole
   B. metronidazole
   C. clotrimazole
   D. ketaconazole

222. What is the trade name for famotidine?
    A. PEPCID
    B. PROPULSID
    C. PRILOSEC
    D. AXID

223. Serotonin-type antidepressants are contraindicated in patients treated with which of the following?
    A. NSAIDs
    B. MAO inhibitors
    C. proton pump inhibitors
    D. HMG-CoA reductase inhibitors

224. Which of the following is the generic name for GLUCOTROL?
    A. glyburide
    B. tolbutamide
    C. glucagon
    D. glipizide

225. Coadministration of verapamil and which of the following may produce an unwanted result?
    A. quinidine
    B. carbamazapine
    C. cimetidine
    D. all of the above

226. Which of the following best describes the drug class for azathioprine?
    A. cardiovascular agents
    B. anticonvulsant drugs
    C. nonsteroidal anti-inflammatory agents
    D. immunosuppressive agents

227. What notable information should you know about ondansetron?
    A. All forms of the medication must be kept in the refrigerator.
    B. Maximum daily dose of 8 mg is used to PREVENT and not to TREAT nausea and vomiting.

C. Give dose 30 minutes before chemotherapy dosing.
    D. B and C

228. Which of the following answers best describes the most common indication for nifedipine?
    A. depression
    B. gastric hypersecretion
    C. angina
    D. myocardial infarction

229. Hydantoin anticonvulsant agents are contraindicated in patients treated with which of the following?
    A. cyclosporine
    B. bumetanide
    C. glipizide
    D. sucralfate

230. Which of the following is a common side effect reported with digoxin use?
    A. loss of appetite
    B. hair loss
    C. excessive hair growth
    D. coating on the tongue

231. The usual adult dose for nafcillin is
    A. 500 mg–1 gm q12h IV
    B. 1–2 gm q4h IV
    C. 1–2 gm q24h IV
    D. 1–2 gm q6h po

232. What information should you give the patient taking naproxen?
    A. Do not take more than 10 days for pain without physician approval.
    B. Double up on missed doses.
    C. Decrease dose if stools are blackened.
    D. Rise slowly from a seated or lying position.

233. While taking captopril, special care should be taken to monitor concurrent use of which of the following drugs?
   A. potassium-sparing diuretics
   B. NSAIDs
   C. oral contraceptives
   D. muscle relaxants

234. Which of the following drugs is commonly used during code blue or cardiac arrest situations?
   A. heparin
   B. losartan
   C. atenolol
   D. epinephrine

235. Carbamazepine anticonvulsant agent is contraindicated in patients treated with which of the following?
   A. macrolide antibiotics
   B. propoxyphene analgesics
   C. saline laxatives
   D. A and B

236. Coadministration of paroxetine and which of the following may result in a potentially serious or even life-threatening drug interaction?
   A. salt replacement products
   B. MAO inhibitors
   C. ethanolamine antihistamines
   D. fluoroquinolones

237. Which of the following is a trade name for insulin?
   A. DIABETA
   B. MICRONASE
   C. GLUCOTROL
   D. HUMULIN

238. Which is an appropriate auxiliary label to use with diclofenac?
   A. Take on an empty stomach.

B. Take with food or milk.
   C. Do not take dairy products or antacid preparations within one hour of this medication.
   D. Finish all this medication unless otherwise directed by prescriber.

239. What is the generic name for the drug DILANTIN?
   A. primidone
   B. phenytoin
   C. valproic acid
   D. mephenytoin

240. If gentamicin is being given to a patient, which drug could help increase the risk of nephrotoxicity if co-administered with gentamicin?
   A. amphoterecin B
   B. metoprolol
   C. insulin
   D. heparin

241. Anticoagulant agents are contraindicated in patients treated with which of the following?
   A. guaifenesin
   B. kaolin/pectin
   C. metronidazole
   D. loperamide

242. Which of the following answers best describes the primary indicated use for digoxin?
   A. PUD
   B. GERD
   C. CHF
   D. NIDDM

243. The main indication for CORVERT is
   A. new onset hypertension
   B. prolonged CHF
   C. asystole
   D. termination of acute a-fib or a-flutter

244. Using the key word "neurotransmission" as the basis for your decision, which of the following does not belong?
    A. sertraline
    B. paroxetine
    C. fluoxetine
    D. cephradine

245. Which of the following drugs does not belong with the others?
    A. CLARITIN
    B. ASTELIN
    C. NASACORT
    D. FLONASE

246. Which is an appropriate auxiliary label to use with levothyroxine?
    A. Avoid smoking while taking this medication.
    B. Use this medication exactly as directed. Do not skip doses or discontinue unless directed by your doctor.
    C. Do not crush.
    D. Take with food or milk.

247. Co-trimoxazole compounds are contraindicated in patients treated with which of the following?
    A. multiple vitamins containing trace elements
    B. anticoagulants
    C. glucocorticosteroids
    D. NSAIDs

248. Coadministration of clonazepam and which of the following may result in a potentially serious or even life-threatening drug interaction?
    A. prednisone
    B. nefazodone
    C. ibuprofen
    D. captopril

249. Using the key acronym "PUD" as the basis for your decision, which of the following does not belong?
    A. nizatidine
    B. famotidine
    C. metronidazole
    D. sucralfate

250. What is the brand name for latanoprost?
    A. COSOPT
    B. XALATAN
    C. TRUSOPT
    D. IOPIDINE

251. Acetazolamide is classified under what drug category?
    A. diuretic (loop)
    B. anticoagulant
    C. diuretic (carbonic anhydrase inhibitor)
    D. diuretic (thiazide-type)

252. Which of the following is the generic name for ROBINUL?
    A. glipizide
    B. glycopyrrolate
    C. glyburide
    D. griseofulvin

253. Benzodiazepines are contraindicated in patients treated with which of the following?
    A. macrolide antibiotics
    B. HMG-CoA reductase inhibitors
    C. bulk laxatives
    D. hormones

254. What class is PERMAX classified into?
    A. antihyperlipidemic
    B. antihypertensive
    C. antiplatelet
    D. anti-Parkinson's disease

255. Which of the following answers best describes the most common indications for conjugated estrogens?
   A. contraception
   B. sexually transmitted disease treatment
   C. estrogen replacement therapy for menopausal symptoms and osteoporosis
   D. conjunctivitis

256. What is the brand name for megestrol?
   A. MEGACE
   B. METFORMIN
   C. MINIPRES
   D. MERREM

257. Which of the following is a common side effect reported with fluconazole use?
   A. rash
   B. flushing
   C. hallucinations
   D. numbness in toes and fingers

258. Coadministration of ibuprofen and which of the following may result in a potentially serious or even life-threatening drug interaction?
   A. fluoxetine
   B. lithium
   C. diphenhydramine
   D. phenytoin

259. How would you classify or group paclitaxel?
   A. antihistamine agent
   B. antiulcer agent
   C. antineoplastic agent
   D. anti-infective agent

260. What is/are the brand names for isosorbide mononitrate?
   A. IMDUR
   B. ISMO

C. ISORDIL
D. A and B

261. Which of the following is the trade name for levothyroxine?
   A. SYMMETREL
   B. SYNALGOS-DC
   C. LEVSIN
   D. SYNTHROID

262. Which of the following is a trade name for potassium chloride?
   A. KAOPECTATE
   B. KLONOPIN
   C. KAY CIEL
   D. KEFLEX

263. Which of the following drug classes or groups is represented by cefaclor?
   A. cardiovascular (beta blocker)
   B. analgesic (opiod)
   C. antibiotic (cephalosporin)
   D. bronchodilator (xanthine)

264. Which of the following medication(s) would you see used in a surgery?
   A. ketamine
   B. midazolam
   C. fentanyl
   D. all of the above

265. Which of the following answers best describes the primary indicated use for ondansetron?
   A. diarrhea resulting from protozoal infestation
   B. migraine headache
   C. emesis associated with emetogenic chemotherapeutic agents
   D. chronic fatigue syndrome

266. Which answer best describes the usual adult dose for lisinopril?

A. up to 40 mcg per day
B. up to 40 mg per day
C. 40 mcg BID
D. 40 mg BID

267. Which of the following is a side effect reported with nizatidine?
A. cough
B. runny nose
C. sweats
D. constipation

268. What principle information should be noted with alprazolam?
A. Avoid alcohol.
B. May cause drug dependence.
C. Discontinue gradually after prolonged use.
D. all of the above

269. Coadministration of conjugated estrogens and which of the following may produce an unwanted result?
A. ibuprofen
B. folic acid
C. tamoxifen
D. nalidixic acid

270. The usual adult dose for hyoscyamine is what?
A. 1 mg qid
B. 0.125 mg tid-qid SL
C. 0.375 mg timed release q12h
D. B and C

271. Which answer best describes the usual adult dose for prazosin?
A. maximum dose of 20 mcg/d
B. minimum dose of 20 mg/d
C. 20 mcg/Kg TID
D. maximum dose of 20 mg/d

272. COLESTID is to colestipol as COLY-MYCIN M is to _____.

A. colfosceril
B. colchicine
C. colistimethate
D. clofibrate

273. Which drug given with lamotrigine would give a drug–drug interaction?
A. valproic acid
B. carbamazepine
C. both A and B
D. none of the above

274. The combination of lidocaine and prilocaine is more commonly known as
A. XYLOCAINE
B. EMLA
C. SENSORCAINE
D. TUCKS PADS

275. Which answer best describes the usual adult oral dose for glyburide?
A. up to 40 mg per day
B. up to 30 mg per day
C. 10 mg TID
D. up to 20 mg per day

276. Which of the following is a side effect reported with levothyroxine?
A. tachycardia
B. nervousness
C. changes in menstrual cycle
D. all of the above

277. What information should you give a patient taking conjugated estrogens?
A. Report unusual bleeding or spotting.
B. Report experiences of depression.
C. Do not take this medication if pregnant or intending to become pregnant.
D. all of the above

278. Which of the following would be prescribed to treat Influenza A?
    A. SYMMETREL
    B. VALTREX
    C. FAMVIR
    D. PRIMAXIN

279. Using the key phrase "birth control" as the basis for your decision, which of the following does not belong?
    A. mestranol/norethindrone
    B. mestranol/norethynodrel
    C. ethinyl estradiol/levonorgestrel
    D. estradiol

280. Which of the following is the trade name for glyburide?
    A. DIABETA
    B. GLYNASE
    C. MICRONASE
    D. all of the above

281. What is the indication of use for the drug REMERON?
    A. treat drowsiness
    B. treat high blood pressure
    C. treat depression
    D. treat Alzheimer's disease

282. Clindamycin is to CLEOCIN as _____ is to CLINORIL?
    A. sulindac
    B. clemastine
    C. sumatriptan
    D. clarithromycin

283. What class is the drug CELLCEPT placed into?
    A. antineoplastic
    B. diuretic
    C. growth hormone
    D. immunosuppressant

284. How would you classify or group nizatidine?
    A. SSRI
    B. histamine H-2 blocker
    C. selective 5-HT-3 receptor blocker
    D. NSAID

285. Which is an appropriate auxiliary label to use with phenytoin?
    A. Take on an empty stomach.
    B. May cause drowsiness.
    C. Do not crush or chew.
    D. Take with plenty of water.

286. Which of the following answers best describes the primary indicated use for diclofenac?
    A. bacterial infection
    B. relieve pain and reduce inflammation
    C. carcinoma
    D. reduce cholesterol level

287. Which answer best describes the usual adult oral dose for digoxin?
    A. up to 0.5 mg per day
    B. 1.5 mg loading dose, 3.0 mg daily thereafter
    C. 0.125 mg qid
    D. 0.25 mg QOD

288. Which of the following is a common side effect reported with diltiazem?
    A. vomiting
    B. nausea
    C. headache
    D. constipation

289. The drug ARTHROTEC has what ingredients in it?
    A. diclofenac and lansoprazole
    B. diclofenac and misoprostol
    C. misoprostol and lansoprazole
    D. misoprostol and ibuprofen

290. Coadministration of fluoxetine and which of the following may produce an unwanted result?
    A. diet high in vitamin K
    B. glipizide
    C. ibuprofen
    D. MAO inhibitors

291. What information should you give a patient taking paroxetine?
    A. A response may take several weeks.
    B. Doses should be adjusted at 7-day intervals.
    C. Take medication with food.
    D. A and B

292. Using the key word "hypertension" as the basis for your decision, which of the following does not belong?
    A. isradipine
    B. diltiazem
    C. enalapril
    D. procainamide

293. What is used as an antidote for benzodiazepine overdose?
    A. naloxone
    B. protamine
    C. flumazenil
    D. charcoal

294. What drug class or group does tacrolimus belong in?
    A. antibiotic
    B. volume expander
    C. antidiarrheal
    D. immunosuppressant

295. Which of the following answers best describes the primary indicated use for gold sodium thiomalate?
    A. delayed puberty
    B. neurogenic diabetes insipidus
    C. inhibited growth
    D. rheumatoid arthritis

296. What is the generic name for ZOSYN?
    A. piperacillin and tazobactam
    B. piperacillin
    C. ticarcillin and clavulanate
    D. ampicillin and sulbactam

297. Coadministration of phenytoin and which of the following may result in a potentially serious or even life-threatening drug interaction?
    A. loperamide
    B. ipratropium
    C. cimetidine
    D. penicillin

298. Which of the following drugs can be given sublingually, buccally, topically, and transdermally?
    A. furosemide
    B. ondansetron
    C. nitroglycerin
    D. dopamine

299. Which is an appropriate strip label to use with naproxen?
    A. Take with food or milk.
    B. Take on an empty stomach.
    C. Avoid exposure to sunlight.
    D. none of the above

300. Coadministration of methotrexate and which of the following may result in a potentially serious or even life-threatening drug interaction?
    A. analgesics
    B. ACE inhibitors
    C. NSAIDs
    D. antispasmodics

301. The "pril" in the names of captopril, enalapril, lisinopril, and ramipril best describes these drugs as which of the following?
  A. calcium channel blockers
  B. ACE inhibitors
  C. inotropics
  D. beta-adrenergic blockers

302. What is the generic name for cromolyn sodium?
  A. NASALCROM
  B. PROVENTIL
  C. BECONASE
  D. FLOVENT

303. Using the key phrase "cardiac arrhythmias" as the basis for your decision, which of the following does not belong?
  A. quinidine
  B. diphenhydramine
  C. procainamide
  D. diphenylhydantoin

304. Which of the following drugs is a protease inhibitor?
  A. acyclovir
  B. stavudine
  C. zidovudine
  D. indinavir

305. Which of the following answers best describes the primary indicated use for hydroxychloroquine?
  A. malaria
  B. muscle spasm
  C. depression
  D. myocardial infarction

306. Which answer best describes the usual adult dose for naproxen?
  A. 1.5 g/d
  B. 1.5 mg/d

  C. 1.5 mcg QID
  D. 1.5 g BID

307. Which of the following is a common side effect reported with furosemide?
  A. vomiting
  B. orthostatic hypotension
  C. nausea
  D. dehydration

308. What information should you give a patient taking nizatidine?
  A. Avoid aspirin.
  B. Avoid black pepper, caffeine, and harsh spices.
  C. Avoid alcohol.
  D. all of the above

309. The OTC medication Tavist-1 contains what ingredient?
  A. diphenhydramine
  B. tripolidine
  C. clemestine
  D. chlorpheniramine

310. Coadministration of medroxyprogesterone and which of the following may produce an unwanted result?
  A. aminoglutethimide
  B. bumetamide
  C. chlorpropamide
  D. desonide

311. Which answer best describes the usual adult dose for pravastatin?
  A. 40 mg TID
  B. up to 40 mg/day
  C. 40 mcg/kg/d in divided dose
  D. up to 40 mcg once a day

312. Using the key words "calcium channel blocker" as the basis for your decision, which of the following does not belong?
  A. metoprolol

B. felodipine

C. bepridil

D. diltiazem

313. Which of the following is the trade name for naproxen?
    A. NAPROSYN
    B. ANAPROX
    C. NALFON
    D. A and B

314. What information should you give a patient taking enalapril?
    A. Report a persistent cough.
    B. Do not crush tablets.
    C. Take medication with food or milk.
    D. Take medication on an empty stomach.

315. Which of the following answers best describes the primary indicated use for furosemide?
    A. dermatitis
    B. edema
    C. arrhythmia
    D. none of the above

316. In what class does the drug vecuronium belong?
    A. antispasmodic
    B. neuromuscular blocking agent
    C. antidepressant
    D. non-narcotic analgesic agent

317. Which answer best describes the usual adult dose for nizatidine?
    A. 300 mcg qhs
    B. 300 mg BID
    C. up to 300 mg/day
    D. 30 mg prn

318. Which of the following is a side effect reported with gold sodium thiomalate?

A. metallic taste

B. tongue irritation

C. oral ulcers

D. all of the above

319. Which is an appropriate auxiliary label to use with nizatidine?
    A. Avoid prolonged exposure to sunlight.
    B. May cause drowsiness.
    C. Take on an empty stomach.
    D. Protect medication from light.

320. Minocycline should not be given with which of the following drugs?
    A. diuretics
    B. laxatives
    C. antacids
    D. antihypertensives

321. The "dipine" in the names of felodipine, isradipine, nicardipine, nifedipine, and nimodipine best describes these drugs as which of the following?
    A. ACE inhibitors
    B. calcium channel blockers
    C. beta-adrenergic blockers
    D. alpha-adrenergic blockers

322. How often should a fentanyl patch be changed?
    A. once a week
    B. once a month
    C. once a day
    D. once every 3 days

323. Which is a brand name for nifedipine?
    A. PROCAN
    B. PROCARDIA
    C. PRINVIL
    D. PROVENTIL

324. Which of the following drugs would you use to induce vomiting in cases of overdosing?
   A. charcoal
   B. ipecac
   C. promethazine
   D. trimethobenzamide

325. EPSOM SALT contains which of the following?
   A. magnesium sulfate
   B. magnesium oxide
   C. magnesium hydroxide
   D. magnesium citrate

326. Which of the following is the trade name for warfarin?
   A. CALAN
   B. WYDASE
   C. COUMADIN
   D. CAPOTEN

327. Amlodipine is to NORVASC as _____ is to NAVANE.
   A. amoxapine
   B. thiothixene
   C. amitriptyline
   D. thioridazine

328. Which of the following is a side effect reported with ibuprofen?
   A. diarrhea
   B. heartburn
   C. constipation
   D. irritability

329. Which of the following answers best describes the primary indicated use for paclitaxel?
   A. malignant prostate cancer
   B. lymphoma
   C. testicular carcinoma
   D. carcinoma of the ovaries and breast

330. The purpose of choral hydrate is for use as a
   A. sedative
   B. antibiotic
   C. mineral supplement
   D. diuretic

331. Coadministration of lovastatin and which of the following may result in a potentially life-threatening drug interaction?
   A. macrolide antibiotics
   B. cholesterol drugs
   C. transplant drugs
   D. all of the above

332. Using the key word "inotropic" as the basis for your decision, which of the following does not belong?
   A. digitoxin
   B. metronidazole
   C. dosoxin
   D. milrinone

333. Which of the following is the trade name for silver sulfadiazine?
   A. THERMAZENE
   B. SILVADENE
   C. BACTRIM
   D. both A and B

334. What is the generic name for BETADINE?
   A. povidone
   B. hexachlorophene
   C. povidone-iodine
   D. iodine

335. Which answer best describes the usual adult dose for propoxyphene napsylate/acetaminophen?
   A. starting dose of 100 mg titrated up until pain is relieved
   B. maximum up to 600 mg/day

C. 600 mcg qhs

D. 60 mg/kg q6h

336. How would you classify or group insulin?

A. immunosuppressive agent

B. hypoglycemic agent

C. osteoporosis agent

D. colony stimulating factor

337. Which of the following answers best describes the most common indication for cefaclor?

A. major depression

B. seasonal affective disorder

C. infection caused by susceptible organisms

D. ulcers

338. What ingredients are in the product COMBIVENT?

A. albuterol and salmeterol

B. albuterol and ipratropium

C. ipratropium and salmeterol

D. albuterol and fluticasone

339. What information should you give the patient taking diltiazem?

A. Discontinue gradually.

B. Double the dose if you feel your heart pounding.

C. Crush the sustained release form if you cannot swallow it whole.

D. none of the above

340. Which of the following is the generic name for MICRONASE?

A. glipizide

B. glyburide

C. tolazamide

D. tolbutamide

341. Which of the following is a side effect reported with paroxetine?

A. ejaculatory disturbance

B. increased pulse rate

C. fever

D. yellowing skin

342. Using the key word "antineoplastic" as the basis for your decision, which of the following does not belong?

A. cyclophosphamide

B. etoposide

C. allopurinol

D. melphalan

343. Which of the following is the trade name for diclofenac?

A. VOSOL

B. DIDRONEL

C. VOLTAREN

D. VIVACTIL

344. What is the generic name for the drug LANOXIN?

A. digoxin

B. digitoxin

C. diphenhydramine

D. propranolol

345. The product SELSUN contains what ingredient?

A. silicon dioxide

B. minoxidil

C. selenium sulfide

D. hexachlorophene

346. Which is an appropriate strip label to use with diltiazem?

A. Take with milk or food.

B. This medication may impair the ability to drive or operate machinery.

C. Take with a full glass of water.

D. May cause discoloration of the urine or feces.

347. Which is an appropriate auxiliary label to use with potassium chloride?
   A. Swallow tablets whole.
   B. Dilute before using (liquid form).
   C. Protect from light.
   D. A and B

348. Which answer best describes the usual adult dose for lovastatin?
   A. maximum 8 gm/day
   B. 80 mcg qd
   C. 40 mg qd
   D. maximum 80 mg/day

349. Which of the following is a side effect reported with insulin?
   A. hair loss
   B. loss of memory
   C. sweating
   D. metallic taste

350. What is CORLOPAM indicated for?
   A. Parkinson's disease
   B. severe hypertension
   C. hair loss
   D. depression

351. What is the trade or brand name for the generic drug amoxicillin?
   A. OMNIPEN
   B. UNASYN
   C. ERYTHROCIN
   D. AMOXIL

352. How would you classify or group LO-MOTIL?
   A. antiemetic agent
   B. antidiarrheal agent
   C. anticonvulsant
   D. antihyperlipidemic agent

353. What information should you give a patient taking phenytoin?

   A. Use the same manufacturer's brand of drug.
   B. Take medication with food.
   C. Medication may cause drowsiness.
   D. all of the above

354. What information should you give a patient taking fluconazole?
   A. Complete the full course of therapy.
   B. Do not chew or crush the medication.
   C. Visual disturbances are common, but not dangerous.
   D. Increase your dietary fiber.

355. Which of the following answers best describes the usual dosage for cefaclor?
   A. children: no dose under 12 years old; adult: 500 mg BID
   B. children: 250 mg TID; adults: 500 mg TID
   C. children and adult dose are the same
   D. children: up to 40 mg/kg/day divided every 8–12 hours; adults: 250–500 mg q8h

356. Which of the following is a side effect reported with ketorolac?
   A. loss of appetite
   B. joint pain
   C. loss of muscle coordination
   D. drowsiness

357. What information should you give a patient taking omeprazole?
   A. Take medication before eating.
   B. Swallow medication whole.
   C. Do not chew, crush, or break medication.
   D. all of the above

358. Long-term concurrent use of acetaminophen and which of the following poses a potential threat for liver damage?
   A. alcohol

B. anticonvulsant drugs

C. tuberculosis drugs

D. all of the above

359. Coadministration of potassium chloride and which of the following may result in a potentially serious or even life-threatening drug interaction?

A. hypoglycemic drugs

B. potassium-sparing diuretics

C. laxatives

D. antigout drugs

360. Using the key word "inflammation" as the basis for your decision, which of the following does not belong?

A. diflunisal

B. fluconazole

C. fenoprofen

D. diclofenac

361. How would you classify or group lisinopril?

A. inotropic agent

B. calcium channel blocker

C. ACE inhibitor

D. beta-adrenergic blocker

362. How would you classify or group gold sodium thiomalate?

A. nonsteroidal anti-inflammatory agent

B. osteoporosis agent

C. rheumatoid arthritic agent

D. skeletal growth factor

363. What information should you give the patient taking sertraline?

A. Dose changes may be made at 1-week intervals.

B. Males may experience sexual dysfunction.

C. An observable response may take several weeks.

D. all of the above

364. Which of the following is the trade name for diltiazem?

A. CARDIZEM

B. TENORMIN

C. ISOPTIN

D. PLENDIL

365. Using the key word "electrolyte" as the basis for your decision, which of the following does not belong?

A. sodium chloride

B. copper sulfate

C. calcium gluconate

D. potassium chloride

366. Which of the following is a side effect reported with nabumetone?

A. blurred vision

B. heartburn

C. weakness

D. thirst

367. What information should you give a patient taking glipizide?

A. Do not skip meals.

B. Do not take double doses.

C. Avoid OTC cough/cold, appetite control, hay fever, and asthma preparations.

D. all of the above

368. Coadministration of insulin and which of the following may produce an unwanted result?

A. corticosteroids

B. thyroid hormones

C. oral contraceptives

D. all of the above

369. Using the key word "hormone" as the basis for your decision, which of the following does not belong?

A. methyltestosterone

B. methylprednisolone

C. insulin

D. estrogen

370. A representative of the histamine H-2 receptor antagonist class of drugs is which of the following?
   A. ranitidine
   B. ipratropium
   C. labetolol
   D. glipizide

371. Using the key phrase "potassium-sparing" as the basis for your decision, which of the following does not belong?
   A. spironolactone
   B. triamterene/hydrochlorothiazide
   C. furosemide
   D. amiloride

372. What information should you give the patient taking digoxin?
   A. Report blood in stools.
   B. Report skin rash.
   C. Report discoloration of the tongue.
   D. Report visual disturbances.

373. Which of the following answers best describes the usual adult oral dosage for clarithromycin?
   A. Duration and dosage depend on the type of infection.
   B. 250 mg TID for 21 days
   C. 500 mg TID for 10–14 days
   D. dosage range between 250–500 mg TID for 14 days

374. Which of the following is a side effect reported with omeprazole?
   A. glossitis
   B. arthralgia
   C. rapid heart rate
   D. changes in bowel movements

375. What is the generic name for the drug ALTACE?
   A. ranitidine
   B. ramipril
   C. rifampin
   D. ritodrine

376. What is the trade name for ondansetron?
   A. ZYLOPRIM
   B. ZOFRAN
   C. ONCOVIN
   D. ZOSYN

377. What information should you give the patient taking lovastatin?
   A. Use medication in conjunction with low-fat dietary restrictions.
   B. Take the medication with a full glass of water.
   C. Maintain a low-salt diet.
   D. Take the medication during the evening.

378. Coadministration of ethinyl estradiol/norethindrone and which of the following may produce an unwanted result?
   A. metoprolol
   B. phenytoin
   C. theophylline
   D. all of the above

379. Using the key word "gout" as the basis for your decision, which of the following does not belong?
   A. colchicine
   B. piroxicam
   C. allopurinol
   D. probenecid

380. Which of the following is the trade name for enalapril?
   A. VASODILAN
   B. VASOCIDIN
   C. VASCOR
   D. VASOTEC

381. Which is an appropriate auxiliary label to use with hydroxychloroquine?

A. Take with food or milk.

B. Avoid smoking while taking this medication.

C. Do not crush.

D. Take on an empty stomach.

382. Which of the following answers best describes the primary indicated use for glipizide?

A. noninsulin-dependent diabetes mellitus

B. insulin-dependent diabetes mellitus

C. juvenile diabetes

D. none of the above

383. Which is an appropriate strip label to use with DILANTIN?

A. Take on an empty stomach.

B. Avoid prolonged exposure to sunlight.

C. Take with food.

D. B and C

384. Which of the following answers best describes the usual oral dosage for conjugated estrogens?

A. 0.3 mg twice a day

B. up to 30 mg daily depending on indication

C. the highest dose tolerated for 20 days

D. 1.25 mg daily for 7 days, followed by 0.625 mg for 21 days

385. Which is an appropriate auxiliary label to use with omeprazole?

A. May cause drowsiness.

B. Do not crush. Swallow whole.

C. May cause discoloration of urine or feces.

D. Avoid prolonged exposure to sunlight.

386. Allopurinol given with which of the following drug groups may precipitate a potentially fatal reaction called the Stevens-Johnson syndrome?

A. ACE inhibitors

B. corticosteroids

C. serotonin reuptake inhibitors

D. diuretics

387. Which of the following answers best describes a unique association with fluoxetine?

A. This medication is used as an adjunct to TCAs.

B. An observable response may take several weeks.

C. The drug has an extremely high safety profile.

D. The effectiveness of this medication can be measured only through blood tests.

388. Using the key word "seizures" as the basis for your decision, which of the following does not belong?

A. doxazosin

B. clonazepam

C. phenytoin

D. valparoic acid

389. The term INTRALIPIDS is also known as what?

A. dextrose

B. saline

C. fat emulsions

D. proteins

390. What is the generic name for AXID?

A. nifedipine

B. nizatidine

C. niacin

D. azathioprine

391. Amitriptyline is to aminophylline as _____ is to bronchodilator.

A. antibiotic

B. antineoplastic

C. antihypertensive

D. antidepressant

392. Which of the following is a primary indication/use for colchicine, while hypercholesterolemia is the primary indication/use for the similarly sounding drug, colestipol?
    A. gouty arthritis
    B. viral infection
    C. diarrhea
    D. migraine

393. Protamine sulfate is to heparin as _____ is to digoxin.
    A. digibind
    B. digitoxin
    C. diltiazem
    D. phytanodione

394. Which of the following is a side effect reported with lisinopril?
    A. cough
    B. itching
    C. nausea and vomiting
    D. excessive thirst

395. The drug ergocalciferol is also known as what?
    A. vitamin A
    B. vitamin C
    C. vitamin D
    D. vitamin E

396. What information should you give the patient taking levothyroxin?
    A. Take each dose with a full glass of orange juice.
    B. The drug may cause drowsiness.
    C. Noticeable effects may take a few weeks.
    D. Double up on missed doses.

397. Which of the following drugs can potentially interact with azathioprine?
    A. propranolol
    B. haloperidol

    C. allopurinol
    D. terconazole

398. QUINAMM is to QUINORA as _____ is to quinidine.
    A. quinapril
    B. quinacrine
    C. quinine
    D. quazepam

399. Which answer best describes the usual adult dose for ranitidine?
    A. 300 mg daily
    B. 300 mg BID
    C. 150 mg TID
    D. 150 mg QID

400. What test antigens are included in an anergy panel or anergy testing kit?
    A. candida albicans skin test antigen, mumps skin test antigen, tuberculin test
    B. candida albicans skin test antigen, poison ivy skin test antigen, histoplasmin
    C. coccidioidin, histoplasmin, contact dermatitis skin test antigen, tuberculin test
    D. candida albicans skin test antigen, mumps skin test antigen, electrical skin test antigen

401. How often should propofol and its tubing be changed out?
    A. every 24 hours
    B. every 12 hours
    C. every 48 hours
    D. every 6 hours

402. Which is an appropriate auxiliary label to use with insulin?
    A. Refrigerate and shake well before using.
    B. For external use only.
    C. Take on an empty stomach 1 hour before or 2 to 3 hours after a meal.
    D. Dilute before administration.

403. What information should you give a patient taking insulin?
    A. Do not use if there are clumps in the insulin after mixing or if bottle has a frosted appearance.
    B. Exercise may lower your need for insulin.
    C. Illness may cause your insulin requirements to change.
    D. all of the above

404. Which is an appropriate strip label to use with digoxin?
    A. May cause discoloration of urine or feces.
    B. Take with plenty of water.
    C. Drink a full glass of orange juice or eat a banana daily while taking this medication.
    D. Take with food or milk.

405. Which of the following is a side effect reported with phenytoin?
    A. slurred speech
    B. insomnia
    C. excessive thirst
    D. excessive sweating

406. Histamine H-2 receptor antagonists are used to treat which of the following conditions?
    A. asthma
    B. diabetes
    C. hypertension
    D. gastric ulcers

407. Which of the following answers best describes the primary indicated use for nizatidine?
    A. joint inflammation
    B. duodenal ulcer
    C. urinary burning
    D. constipation

408. Which of the following is a side effect reported with ketoprofen?
    A. muscle cramps
    B. numbness
    C. indigestion
    D. sore throat

409. Which is an appropriate auxiliary label to use with ketorolac?
    A. Avoid smoking while taking this medication.
    B. May cause drowsiness or dizziness.
    C. Do not crush.
    D. Discard unused portion.

410. Which is an appropriate auxiliary label to use with prazosin?
    A. Take after meals.
    B. May cause drowsiness or dizziness.
    C. Take on an empty stomach.
    D. Avoid prolonged exposure to sunlight.

411. Coadministration of diclofenac and which of the following may produce an unwanted result?
    A. hormones
    B. laxatives
    C. thiazides
    D. vasodilators

412. Which drug is not a platelet inhibitor?
    A. ticlopidine
    B. ranitidine
    C. abciximab
    D. aspirin

413. Which of the following drugs could be given for coughing?
    A. benzoyl peroxide
    B. bumetanide
    C. benzodiazepines
    D. benzonatate

414. What information should you give a patient taking ibuprofen?
    A. Report prolonged heartburn and abdominal pain.
    B. Double up on missed doses.
    C. Medication may cause drowsiness; therefore, test reaction to drug before operating a vehicle.
    D. A and C

415. What information should you give a patient taking potassium chloride?
    A. Do not use salt substitutes while on this medication.
    B. Dissolve the liquid, powder, and effervescent tablet forms in water or juice, and drink slowly.
    C. There is no concern for wax coating from some tablets that may be found in stool.
    D. all of the above

416. Which of the following is the generic name for FOLEX?
    A. metaproterenol
    B. folic acid
    C. methotrexate
    D. flutamide

417. Which of the following drug classes or groups is represented by digoxin?
    A. antihistamine
    B. ACE inhibitor
    C. cardiovascular agent
    D. bronchodilator

418. Which of the following answers best describes the primary indicated use for methotrexate?
    A. leukemias
    B. psoriasis
    C. rheumatoid arthritis
    D. all of the above

419. Which of the following answers best describes a unique association with VANTIN?
    A. Do not freeze liquid preparation.
    B. Entire course of medication is 10–14 days.
    C. Take medication in equal intervals around the clock.
    D. all of the above

420. Coadministration of pravastatin and which of the following may result in a potentially serious or even life-threatening drug interaction?
    A. pseudoephedrine
    B. docusate sodium
    C. gemfibrozil
    D. acetaminophen

421. What is the usual starting dose of dopamine?
    A. 1–5 mcg/kg/min
    B. >20 mcg/kg/min
    C. 5 mcg/hr
    D. 20 mcg/hr

422. Which of the following is not an available strength for SINEMET?
    A. 25/100
    B. 10/100
    C. 75/200
    D. 50/200

423. Coadministration of famotidine and which of the following may produce an unwanted result?
    A. itraconazole
    B. ketaconazole
    C. glycopyrrolate
    D. A and B

424. All of the following will need a loading dose before starting the maintenance dose except

A. phenytoin

B. diltiazem

C. heparin

D. metoclopramide

425. Which of the following is a primary use for clonazepam, while generalized anxiety and panic disorder is the primary indication for the similarly sounding drug, clorazepate?

A. obsessive–compulsive disorder

B. peptic ulcer disease

C. seizures

D. inflammation

426. What is the available dosage form for paclitaxel?

A. IM

B. SQ

C. IV

D. PO

427. Which of the following is a side effect reported with ranitidine?

A. rapid heart rate

B. nausea

C. malaise

D. muscle cramps

428. Which of the following answers best describes a unique association with diltiazem?

A. Medication causes metallic taste.

B. Do not crush the sustained release form of the drug.

C. Avoid antacids while taking this drug.

D. Medication causes urine to change color.

429. Which of the following answers best describes a unique association with digoxin?

A. Chills indicate toxicity.

B. Blood in stools indicates toxicity.

C. Visual disturbances indicate toxicity.

D. Loss of coordination indicates toxicity.

430. Which of the following drugs would be used for prostate cancer?

A. NOLVADEX

B. EULEXIN

C. VIAGRA

D. WELLCOVORIN

431. Which of the following drug classes or groups is represented by amoxicillin?

A. antibiotic agent (beta-lactams)

B. antibiotic agent (tetracyclines)

C. antibiotic agent (fluoroquinolones)

D. antibiotic agent (sulfonamides)

432. Which of the following answers describes an indicated use for medroxyprogesterone?

A. contraception

B. endometrial carcinoma

C. leukemia

D. organ transplant

433. Which of the following drugs is most often prescribed QD?

A. ampicillin capsules

B. carisoprodol tablets

C. digoxin tablets

D. acetaminophen tablets

434. Which of the following answers best describes a unique association with enalapril?

A. causes metallic taste

B. turns urine orange

C. Antacids reduce effectiveness.

D. Discontinue use during second and third trimesters of pregnancy.

435. How would you classify or group potassium chloride?

A. intravenous additive

B. vitamin

C. electrolyte

D. trace element

436. Which of the following is a common side effect reported with glipzide use?
    A. musculoskeletal disturbances
    B. respiratory disturbances
    C. depression
    D. gastrointestinal disturbances

437. Coadministration of digoxin and which of the following may produce an unwanted result?
    A. potassium-sparing diuretics
    B. potassium-wasting diuretics
    C. analgenics
    D. cough suppressants

438. What accounts for the way amlodipine works?
    A. The drug prevents sodium overload.
    B. The drug dilates coronary vessels by relaxing the smooth muscles of the coronary vessels.
    C. The drug balances the elimination and reuptake of sodium, potassium, and calcium.
    D. The drug slows the pumping action of the heart.

439. Which of the following is not a strength that insulin comes as?
    A. 75/25
    B. 70/30
    C. 50/50
    D. none of the above

440. Which of the following answers best describes the primary indicated use for phenytoin?
    A. seasonal affective disorder
    B. hypertension
    C. ulcers
    D. tonic-clonic (grand mal) seizures

441. Which of the following answers best describes a unique association with sertraline?

    A. Refrain from drinking alcohol while taking this drug.
    B. Clean container before instilling dose to each eye.
    C. Take with a full glass of water.
    D. Causes hypotension.

442. If you see an order for a Z-PACK, what drug are you dispensing?
    A. zidovudine
    B. azithromycin
    C. methylprednisolone
    D. zolpidem

443. Which of the following drugs is an HMG-CoA reductase inhibitor?
    A. albuterol
    B. atenolol
    C. glyburide
    D. simvastatin

444. What is the brand name for fluticasone?
    A. FLONASE
    B. BECONASE
    C. FLOVENT
    D. BOTH A AND C

445. Which answer best describes the usual adult dose for sertraline?
    A. 25 mcg qhs
    B. maximum 200 mg/day
    C. 20 mg/kg BID
    D. up to 200 mcg/day

446. _____ is to alprazolam as ZANTAC is to XANAX.
    A. allopurinol
    B. alteplase
    C. ramipril
    D. ranitidine

447. Which of the following best describes a unique association with lovastatin?

A. Exempted from childproof containers.

B. low-salt diet

C. Take with evening meal.

D. Take with plenty of fluid.

448. SOMA COMPOUND contains what two ingredients?

A. carisoprodol/aspirin

B. carisoprodol/aceteminophen

C. carisoprodol/ibuprofen

D. carisoprodol/naproxen

449. Which of the following is a common side effect reported with glyburide use?

A. insomnia

B. gastrointestinal disturbances

C. hair loss

D. depression

450. Which of the following is a side effect reported with potassium chloride?

A. flatulence

B. oral ulcers

C. salty taste

D. bruising

451. Beta-blockers may mask signs and symptoms of what disease?

A. migraines

B. arthritis

C. diabetes

D. gout

452. Which of the following answers best describes the primary indicated use for TOPROL XL?

A. COPD

B. hypertension

C. CHF

D. anxiety

453. What is the generic name for the drug ACTOS?

A. glimepiride

B. acarbose

C. pioglitazone

D. miglitol

454. Which of the following answers best describes a unique association with omeprazole?

A. Causes urine discoloration.

B. Must be swallowed whole.

C. Take medication with plenty of fluid.

D. Store in glass.

455. Which is an appropriate auxiliary label to use with fluoxetine?

A. Take on a full stomach.

B. May cause drowsiness.

C. Take on an empty stomach.

D. May cause discoloration of urine or feces.

456. Which of the following answers best describes the most common indication for ciprofloxacin?

A. hepatitis

B. infection caused by susceptible strains of organisms

C. endocarditis

D. viral infection of the upper respiratory tract

457. What is the usual adult dose for ZOSYN?

A. 2.25 gm IV q6h

B. 3.375 gm IV q24h

C. 2.25 gm IV q12h

D. 3.375 gm IV q6h

458. Which of the following answers best describes the usual adult oral dosage for captopril?

A. maximum dose: 450 mg per day

B. maximum dose: 50 mg QID

C. dose range: 50–200 mg

D. dose range: 25–100 mg

459. Which of the following is a side effect reported with nisoldipine?
   A. dry mouth
   B. fever
   C. headaches
   D. drowsiness

460. What information should you give a patient taking hydroxychloroquine?
   A. Complete the full course of therapy.
   B. Protect eyes from sunlight.
   C. Report ringing in the ears (tinnitus).
   D. all of the above

461. Coadministration of glyburide and which of the following may produce an unwanted result?
   A. NSAIDs
   B. salicylates
   C. thiazides
   D. all of the above

462. What information should you give a patient taking pravastatin?
   A. Use in conjunction with dietary therapy.
   B. Take medication only after eating high-fat meals.
   C. Take a blood test for lipid profile every 3 weeks.
   D. Double dose if a dose is missed.

463. Which of the following answers best describes a unique association with conjugated estrogens?
   A. Use of medication is restricted to osteoporosis in elderly patients.
   B. Avoid alcohol.
   C. Do not use during pregnancy.
   D. Chew tablets before swallowing.

464. DYNACIRC is to hypertension as GLUCOVANCE is to _____.

   A. Parkinson's disease
   B. diabetes
   C. Alzheimer's disease
   D. depression

465. LUPRON DEPOT KIT is used for what disease?
   A. growth hormone
   B. fertility agent
   C. advanced pancreatic cancer
   D. advanced prostate carcinoma

466. Coadministration of prazosin and which of the following may produce an unwanted result?
   A. verapamil
   B. codeine
   C. prednisone
   D. ergotamine

467. PERSANTINE is to PLAVIX as VIOXX is to _____.
   A. VANCOCIN
   B. CELEBREX
   C. VANTIN
   D. CELEXA

468. Which of the following drug classes or groups is represented by amikacin?
   A. anti-infectives (beta-lactams)
   B. anti-infectives (aminoglycosides)
   C. anti-infectives (cephalosporins)
   D. anti-infectives (macrolides)

469. What best describes a unique association with warfarin sodium?
   A. May cause a change in urine color.
   B. Should be taken with food.
   C. Causes a metallic taste.
   D. Double up missed doses.

470. Donepezil can lead to a drug interaction with which of the following?
    A. phenytoin
    B. quinidine
    C. carbamazepine
    D. all of the above

471. Which of the following is the generic name for MINIPRESS?
    A. pravastatin
    B. minoxidil
    C. propofol
    D. prazosin

472. Which of the following is a side effect reported with lovastatin?
    A. excessive thirst
    B. flatus
    C. chills
    D. wheezing

473. Which of the following answers best describes a unique association with amoxicillin?
    A. Take drug with food to reduce gastric upset.
    B. Avoid antacids while taking drug.
    C. Take drug around the clock in equal intervals.
    D. Store drug in glass container.

474. What information should you give a patient taking loratadine?
    A. Drink fluid liberally.
    B. Reduce coffee consumption while taking this medication.
    C. Take medication with a full glass of orange juice.
    D. Double up on missed doses.

475. Pramoxine is to hemorrhoids as silver sulfadiazine is to _____.

    A. warts
    B. burns
    C. inflammation
    D. red eye

476. Coadministration of loratadine and which of the following may produce an unwanted result?
    A. calcium channel blocking agents
    B. triazole antifungal agents
    C. laxatives
    D. antiemetic agents

477. Protease inhibitors are used primarily to treat which of the following conditions?
    A. HIV infection
    B. asthma
    C. diabetes
    D. hyperlipidemia

478. What is the usual starting adult dose for venlafaxine extended-release?
    A. 75 mg per day with food
    B. 150 mg per day without food
    C. 75 mg q8h with food
    D. 7.5 mg per day with food

479. Which of the following answers best describes the primary indicated use for potassium chloride?
    A. hyponatremia
    B. hyperkalemia
    C. hypoglycemia
    D. hypokalemia

480. DEMADEX is to LASIX as TRANDATE is to _____.
    A. DILTIAZEM
    B. CATAPRES
    C. LOPRESSOR
    D. WYTENSIN

481. Which of the following drug classes or groups is represented by diltiazem?
    A. analgesic agent (opioid)
    B. anti-infective agent (beta-lactam)
    C. cardiovascular agent (calcium channel blocker)
    D. hormone agent (anabolic steroid)

482. The generic name for ROBINUL is what?
    A. glipizide
    B. gabapentin
    C. gancyclovir
    D. glycopyrrolate

483. MACRODANTIN can interact with which of the following?
    A. nisoldipine
    B. amoxicillin
    C. antacids
    D. glyburide

484. What is the usual dose for an adult when prescribing TRENTAL?
    A. 400 mg qd
    B. 400 mg q12h prn
    C. 400 mg tid
    D. 400 mg q48h

485. What is the brand name for phenytoin?
    A. VANTIN
    B. ZARONTIN
    C. NEURONTIN
    D. DILANTIN

486. Which of the following is a side effect reported with medroxyprogesterone?
    A. bleeding
    B. changes in menstrual flow
    C. edema
    D. all of the above

487. Which answer best describes the usual adult dose for simvastatin?

A. up to 40 mg once a day
B. maximum of 40 mcg daily
C. 40 mg in the AM and PM
D. 4 mg qhs

488. BETOPTIC is to TIMOPTIC as betaxolol is to _____.
    A. timolol
    B. tioconazole
    C. carteolol
    D. levobunolol

489. Which of the following is the most common side effect of BRICANYL?
    A. drowsiness
    B. nervousness
    C. dry mouth
    D. urinary incontinence

490. Which of the following answers best describes a unique association with ciprofloxacin?
    A. Avoid antacids containing magnesium or aluminum, or products with iron or zinc within 4 hours before or 2 hours after dosing.
    B. Store medication under refrigerated conditions.
    C. Do not crush or chew medication.
    D. Medication causes a metallic taste.

491. Which is an appropriate strip label to use with ranitidine?
    A. Take with food.
    B. Protect from light.
    C. May cause drowsiness.
    D. May cause discoloration of urine or feces.

492. Coadministration of fluconazole and which of the following may produce an unwanted result?

A. metoprolol

B. methocarbamol

C. diphenhydramine

D. warfarin

493. Which drug prepared parenterally should never be put in a PVC bag?

A. erythromycin

B. dopamine

C. ranitidine

D. paclitaxol

494. The generic name for DESOWEN is

A. betamethasone

B. desonide

C. halcinonide

D. halobetasol

495. What information should you give a patient taking prazosin?

A. Monitor blood pressure regularly.

B. Maintain a low-sodium diet.

C. Rise slowly from a sitting or lying position.

D. all of the above

496. If a patient needs to be induced into vomiting, which of the following would you use to achieve it?

A. promethazine

B. ondansetron

C. bisacodyl

D. ipecac syrup

497. Which of the following best describes a unique association with NEORAL oral solution?

A. It should be mixed with anything else.

B. It can be mixed with orange juice for better taste.

C. It can be interchanged with SANDIM-MUNE if needed.

D. It can only be mixed with water.

498. Which of the following best describes the primary indicated use for levothyroxine?

A. underactive thyroid

B. prevention of pregnancy

C. diabetes insipidus

D. HIV infection

499. Coadministration of propoxyphene napsylate/acetaminophen and which of the following may result in a potentially serious or even life-threatening drug interaction?

A. senna

B. lactulose

C. diphenoxylate

D. carbamazepine

500. Which of the following is an antihistamine that is available in a nasal spray form?

A. chlorpheniramine

B. diphenhydramine

C. azelastine

D. loratidine

501. Which of the following answers best describes the usual oral dosage for medroxyprogesterone?

A. 5 mg daily

B. 10 mg BID

C. dosing dependent on condition being treated

D. none of the above

502. Which of the following is a side effect reported with ZANAFLEX?

A. insomnia

B. headaches

C. daytime sedation

D. nervousness

503. Of the listed answers, which one is a brand name for potassium chloride?
    A. KLONOPIN
    B. K-CLOR
    C. PLENDIL
    D. PRODIUM

504. The primary indication for NORFLEX is which of the following?
    A. muscle relaxant
    B. antibiotic
    C. depression
    D. diuretic

505. CARDURA can interact with which of the following class of drugs?
    A. antibiotics
    B. NSAIDs
    C. anticoagulants
    D. antiepileptics

506. Coadministration of diltiazem and which of the following may produce an unwanted result?
    A. colony stimulating factors
    B. psychotropics
    C. muscle relaxants
    D. beta-blockers

507. Which of the following is the appropriate route of administration for a long-acting penicillin injection?
    A. IV
    B. IM
    C. SQ
    D. subclavian

508. Which of the following is the correct list of ingredients in CORTISPORIN?
    A. neomycin and polymyxin B
    B. neomycin, gramicidin, and hydrocortisone
    C. neomycin, polymyxin B, and hydrocortisone
    D. neomycin, polymyxin B, and prednisolone

509. Which label is appropriate to supplement the regular label on a prescription for conjugated estrogens?
    A. Take with food.
    B. Take on an empty stomach.
    C. May cause drowsiness.
    D. Avoid prolonged exposure to sunlight.

510. Diphenhydramine is to dimenhydrinate as BENADRYL is to _____.
    A. DRAMAMINE
    B. DILANTIN
    C. DYAZIDE
    D. DONNATAL

511. Which of the following drug classes or groups is represented by enalapril?
    A. cardiovascular agent (beta blocker)
    B. cardiovascular agent (diuretic)
    C. cardiovascular agent (ACE inhibitor)
    D. cardiovascular agent (calcium channel blocker)

512. Heparin is to protamine as digoxin is to _____.
    A. naloxone
    B. digoxin immune fab
    C. flumazenil
    D. digitoxin

513. Which of the following answers best describes a unique association with captopril?
    A. Avoid use of drug during second and third trimesters of pregnancy.
    B. Take drug 1 hour before meals.
    C. Drug is found in the milk of nursing mothers.
    D. all of the above

514. Which of the following answers best describes the usual oral dosage for warfarin sodium?
    A. Therapeutic range is 10 mcg/day.
    B. Maintenance dose is between 2–10 mg/day.
    C. Loading dose is 20 mg.
    D. Dose depends on the weight of the patient.

515. Mupirocin is considered a topical _____.
    A. anti-inflammatory agent
    B. anti-itching agent
    C. anti-infective agent
    D. antiviral agent

516. Piroxicam would be to inflammation as propafenone is to _____.
    A. arrythmias
    B. infections
    C. inflammation
    D. ulcers

517. Coadministration of nabumetone and which of the following may result in a potentially serious or even life-threatening drug interaction?
    A. codeine
    B. insulin
    C. glipizide
    D. warfarin

518. What is the trade or brand name for the generic drug clarithromycin?
    A. ERYTHROCIN
    B. BIAXIN
    C. ZITHROMAX
    D. CLEOCIN

519. What special advice can you offer a patient taking aspirin?
    A. Take medication with food or milk to reduce gastric irritation.
    B. Take medication with a full glass of water to reduce gastric irritation.
    C. Finish all the medication unless the prescriber directed differently.
    D. Avoid exposure to sunlight.

520. Which of the following is a side effect reported with prazosin?
    A. arthralgia
    B. orthostatic hypotension
    C. pruritis
    D. urinary retention

521. Which of the following answers best describes a unique association with clarithromycin?
    A. Do not use in pregnant women.
    B. Do not refrigerate suspension.
    C. Do not use a mixed suspension after 14 days.
    D. all of the above

522. Flecainide is to arrythmias as clomipramine is to _____.
    A. hypertension
    B. depression
    C. infection
    D. insomnia

523. Which of the following answers best describes the most common indication for captopril?
    A. angina
    B. hypertension
    C. myocardial infarction
    D. tachycardia

524. What information should you give the patient taking fluoxetine?
    A. Avoid alcohol and alcohol-containing beverages.
    B. Determine the effect of the medication before operating a vehicle.
    C. A response may take several weeks.
    D. all of the above

525. Which is an appropriate auxiliary label to use with lisinopril?
   A. Take with food.
   B. May cause drowsiness or dizziness.
   C. Do not crush. Swallow medication whole.
   D. Avoid exposure to sunlight.

526. Which of the following answers best describes a unique association with phenytoin?
   A. Do not crush medication.
   B. Medication causes hallucinations.
   C. Do not change brands.
   D. Swish oral suspension in mouth before swallowing.

527. Which is an appropriate auxiliary label to use with sertraline?
   A. Do not chew or crush.
   B. Protect medication from light.
   C. Avoid alcohol.
   D. Avoid prolonged exposure to sunlight.

528. Coadministration of levothyroxine and which of the following may produce an unwanted result?
   A. anticoagulants
   B. muscle relaxants
   C. analgesics
   D. laxatives

529. Cefuroxime can interact with which of the following drugs?
   A. psychotherapeutic drugs
   B. oral contraceptive drugs
   C. antiseizure drugs
   D. analgesic drugs

530. Of the following, what should the patient know about taking ranitidine?
   A. A 6:00 PM dosing may be more effective than a bedtime dose because acid secretion increases at around 7:00 PM.
   B. Maintain a low-salt diet for optimum effect.
   C. Store medication in a glass container.
   D. Do not crush or chew the medication.

531. What answer describes a unique association with conjugated estrogens?
   A. Increase vitamin B_6 and folic acid intake while taking this medication.
   B. Increase calcium intake while taking this medication.
   C. This medication renders iron supplements ineffective.
   D. Supplement medication with aspirin to reduce platelet aggregation.

532. What information should you give a patient taking propoxyphene napsylate/acetaminophen?
   A. Rise slowly from a sitting position.
   B. Cigarette smoking decreases effect of the medication.
   C. Avoid alcohol and sedatives while taking this medication.
   D. B and C

533. Which of the following answers best describes a unique association with loratidine?
   A. This medication causes hallucinations.
   B. Drink plenty of water while taking this medication.
   C. Stay out of sunlight while taking this medication.
   D. This medication causes urine discoloration.

534. Which of the following answers best describes the most common indication for clarithromycin?
   A. infection caused by susceptible urinary tract pathogen
   B. infection of bony tissue
   C. infection caused by susceptible respiratory strains of pathogens
   D. infection of the gastrointestinal tract

535. Which of the following answers best describes the usual oral dosage for nifedipine?
    A. titrate adult dosages above 180 mg per day
    B. 120 mg twice a day
    C. adult range between 10–20 mg per day
    D. adult range between 10–20 mg three times a day

536. Coadministration of ethinyl estsradiol/levonorgestrel and which of the following may produce an unwanted result?
    A. codeine
    B. theophylline
    C. guaifenesin
    D. carisoprodol

537. Coadministration of ranitidine and which of the following may produce an unwanted reaction?
    A. cascara sagrada
    B. ketaconazole
    C. phenazopyridine
    D. sertraline

538. What is the brand name for azelastine?
    A. ZELAST
    B. LASTLONG
    C. ASTELIN
    D. HISTALINE

539. What information should you give the patient taking famotidine?
    A. Do not crush tablets.
    B. Once-daily dosing should be taken preferably at bedtime.
    C. Stay out of the sunlight while taking this medication.
    D. Increase ascorbic acid intake while taking this medication.

540. What is the brand name for ketorolac in the ophthalmic form?
    A. TORADOL
    B. STADOL
    C. ACULAR
    D. AGGRENOX

541. What is a usual sign of aspirin overdose?
    A. heart palpitations
    B. tinnitus
    C. diarrhea
    D. throbbing headache

542. THORAZINE is to chlorpromazine as DIABINESE is to _____.
    A. chlorpheniramine
    B. chlorthalidone
    C. chlorprothixene
    D. chlorpropamide

543. Besides treatment of breast carcinomas, what else could MEGACE be used for?
    A. skin cancer
    B. nausea and vomiting
    C. appetite stimulant
    D. hair loss prevention

544. Which answer best describes the primary indicated use for fluconazole?
    A. bacterial infections
    B. candida infections
    C. viral infections
    D. tuberculosis

545. Hydroxyzine is to _____ as ATARAX is to ATIVAN.
    A. lorazepam
    B. diazepam
    C. clonazepam
    D. flurazepam

546. Minocycline should be avoided in what type of patients?
    A. pediatric
    B. geriatric
    C. hypertensive
    D. pregnant

547. What is unique about the preparation and administration of paclitaxel?
    A. Take medication with plenty of fluid.
    B. Do not use with plasticized PVC equipment or devices.
    C. Rinse mouth after each dose.
    D. Protect drug from sunlight.

548. Which of the following is the generic name for KAY CIEL?
    A. sodium chloride
    B. potassium acetate
    C. calcium gluconate
    D. potassium chloride

549. Cephalexin may show a cross-sensitivity to which of the following drugs?
    A. tetracycline
    B. erythromycin
    C. ciprofloxacin
    D. penicillin

550. _____ is to propranolol as ISORDIL is to isosorbide.
    A. IMDUR
    B. IMODIUM
    C. INDERIDE
    D. INDERAL

551. HALCION is to triazolam as RESTORIL is to _____.
    A. diazepam
    B. temazepam
    C. alprazolam
    D. lorazepam

552. Which is an appropriate strip label to use with colchicine?
    A. Take with food or milk.
    B. Avoid alcohol.
    C. Do not take dairy products, antacids, or iron preparations within 1 hour of this medication.
    D. May cause drowsiness.

553. Which best describes a characteristic for clonazepam?
    A. Schedule C-II
    B. Schedule C-III
    C. Schedule C-IV
    D. Schedule C-V

554. What does VOLMAX and VENTOLIN have in common?
    A. Both are names for injectable formulations.
    B. Both are brands for ipratropium.
    C. Both are brands for albuterol.
    D. Both are brands for triamcinolone.

555. Which best describes the primary indicated use for famotidine?
    A. reduces gastric acid secretion
    B. reduces blood cholesterol
    C. reduces fluid retention
    D. stimulates gastric motility

556. Coadministration of cyclophosphamide and _____ may produce an unwanted result.
    A. allopurinol
    B. betamethasone
    C. carisoprodol
    D. diphenhydramine

557. Although cefaclor is absorbed better without food, why may the drug be taken with food?
    A. to reduce stomach upset
    B. to ensure a timely schedule

C. to clinically reduce the absorption rate

D. to make the drug palatable

558. Coadministration of nizatidine and which of the following may produce an unwanted result?

A. nifedipine

B. ketoconazole

C. acetazolamide

D. ramipril

559. Which is an appropriate strip label to use with clonazepam?

A. Take with plenty of water.

B. Take on an empty stomach.

C. Take with food or milk.

D. Avoid alcohol.

560. The generic name for FERGON is what?

A. ferrous sulfate

B. ferrous gluconate

C. ferrous fumarate

D. multivitamin and minerals

561. What is the generic name for the drug DIA-BETA?

A. metformin

B. glyburide

C. glipizide

D. insulin

562. TAPAZOLE is indicated for what condition?

A. depression

B. infection

C. inflammation

D. hyperthyroidism

563. How should cimetidine be taken?

A. Take it with an antacid.

B. Take it on an empty stomach.

C. Take it as a supplement to a proton pump inhibitor.

D. Take it with meals.

564. What would be helpful for a patient taking furosemide to know?

A. Rise slowly from a lying or sitting position.

B. Take medication at bedtime.

C. Take medication early enough during the day to prevent nocturia.

D. A and C

565. What information should you provide a patient taking colchicine?

A. Stop taking drug if GI symptoms occur.

B. Take the drug with nonacidic juice.

C. Continue to take the drug after symptoms have subsided.

D. The 0.5 mg and the 0.6 mg strengths are interchangeable.

566. Calcium acetate is given for what condition?

A. hypocalcemia

B. hyperphosphatemia

C. hypophosphatemia

D. acidosis

567. Which of the following answers best describes the usual oral dosage for amoxicillin?

A. children: 100 mg every 8 hours; adults: up to 500 mg q8h

B. children: 25–100 mg/Kg/d every 8 hours in divided doses; adults: 250–500 mg every 8 hours

C. children: 250 mg BID; adults: 250 mg QID

D. children: 100 mg/Kg every 8 hours; adults: 250 mg per Kg of body weight every 8 hours

568. What is the generic name for NASAL-CROM?
    A. cromolyn sodium
    B. albuterol
    C. fluticasone
    D. cimetidine

569. What is the generic name for PEPCID?
    A. famotidine
    B. lansoprazole
    C. metoclopramide
    D. omeprazole

570. What is the generic name for NASACORT?
    A. fluticasone
    B. beclomethasone
    C. triamcinolone
    D. prednisolone

571. What is the generic name for FELDENE?
    A. sulindac

B. piroxicam
C. cyclobenzaprine
D. carisoprodol

572. What is the generic name for CLINORIL?
    A. sulindac
    B. piroxicam
    C. cyclobenzaprine
    D. carisoprodol

573. What is the generic name for FLEXERIL?
    A. sulindac
    B. piroxicam
    C. cyclobenzaprine
    D. carisoprodol

✓answers & rationales

1.

C. In the question, ergotamine is the generic name and CAFERGOT is the brand name. Therefore, the relationships should be completed by knowing that sucralfate is the generic name of CARAFATE.

2.

C. Enalapril is part of the class of drugs called ACE inhibitors; the drugs in this class are mainly used for hypertension.

3.

A. Ketorolac is the generic name for TORADOL. TOBREX is the brand name for tobramycin, TOFRANIL is the brand name for imipramine, and KYTRIL is the brand name for granisetron.

4.

D. PREMARIN is the brand name for conjugated estrogens. Tamoxifen is a generic name for NOLVADEX; norethindrone and ethinyl estradiol are ingredients in many different birth control pills.

5.

B. ORTHO-NOVUM and NORINYL are brand-name birth control pills. In the second part of the question, the student should realize that diltiazem is a generic name for a hypertensive drug and make the connection to verapamil, another generic-name antihypertensive medication.

6.

D. Fluoxetine is the generic name for PROZAC, a widely used antidepressive medication.

7.

A. HUMULIN is the brand name for insulin. Glipizide is a generic name for GLUCOTROL, glyburide is a generic name for MICRONASE or DIABETA, and chlorpropamide is generic for DIABINESE.

8.

D. Sertraline is generic for ZOLOFT, which is an antidepressant. SSRI is a class of antidepressants and stands for selective serotonin reuptake inhibitor. NSAID means nonsteroidal anti-inflammatory drug, HMG-CoA is for hyperlipidemia, and TCA means tricyclic antidepressants.

9.

C. Penicillin VK is generic for V-CILLIN K. VERELAN is the brand name for verapamil and PENTIDS is an obsolete name for penicillin G, and VISKEN is the brand name for pindolol.

10.

B. Levothyroxin is used to treat hypothyroidism; therefore, it is a thyroid hormone.

11.

A. COUMADIN is the brand name for warfarin. Hydrocortisone is generic for CORTONE, triamcinolone is the generic name for KENALOG, and cortisone is another generic name for CORTONE.

12.

C. Sertraline is an antidepressive also known by the brand name ZOLOFT.

13.

B. Loratidine is a generic name for CLARITIN. ATARAX is the brand name for meclizine, ALLEGRA is the brand name for fexofenadine, and BENADRYL is the brand name for diphenhydramine.

14.

A. Loratidine is CLARITIN; the medication comes as a 10 mg tablet usually given just once a day.

15.

D. Nabumatone is RELAFEN and is an NSAID. Alcohol and aspirin should be avoided because they will increase the chance of GI bleeding and food and/or milk helps to protect the stomach lining and reduce chances of GI bleeding.

16.

D. Ethinyl estradiol/levonorgestrel are an estrogen and progestin combination found in many oral contraceptives.

17.

B. Penicillin VK is an antibiotic and is used to treat infections of mainly gram-positive organisms. The drug has no activity against fungus or protozoan infections.

18.

D. Verapamil should be taken with food due to smaller differences in peak and trough when administered with food. Most sustained release forms of drugs lose the character of sustained release when crushed or dissolved.

19.

C. PRILOSEC is the brand name for omeprazole. Pantoprazole is generic for PROTONIX, lansoparzole is generic for PREVACID, and rabeprezole is generic for ACIPHEX. All are anti-ulcer agents.

20.

D. Colchicine impairs the absorption of vitamin B_{12} by changing the functional capacity of the ileal mucosa, which is a reversible malabsorption syndrome.

21.

A. Nizatidine is AXID. It is available over the counter in a lower dosage strength of 75 mg as compared to 150 mg and 300 mg by prescription.

22.

D. Simvastatin is ZOCOR and is part of the HMG-CoA reductase inhibitor family of antihyperlipidimic drugs. This class is known to cause muscle pain and fever. A patient taking any antihyperlipidimic medication should also incorporate a healthy, low-fat diet in order to get the best results.

23.

D. ADALAT is the brand name for nifedipine. Nisoldipine is generic for SULAR, nizatidine is generic for AXID, and acebutolol is generic for SECTRAL.

24.

C. Fluoxetine is PROZAC and is part of the SSRI family used for depression. Diazepam is a benzodiazepine and is used for anxiety or seizures. Chlorpromazine and haloperidol are classified as antipsychotics.

25.

B. Verapamil is a calcium channel blocker used in the treatment of hypertension and/or angina.

26.

D. Triamterene/hydrochlorothiazide is generic for MAXZIDE and DYAZIDE and is an antihypertensive/diuretic combo. DIUPRES is a brand name for the combo chlorothiazide and reserpine, and DYRENIUM is a brand name for triamterene alone.

27.

B. QUINORA is a brand name for quinidine. Therefore, the correct answer is obtained by realizing that clonidine is a generic name and its corresponding brand name is CATAPRES.

28.

B. Combination of gemfibrozil and simvastatin or any other drug in the "statin" family of antihyperlipidemics can lead to destruction of muscles and increase in potential for renal disease.

29.

D. Ranitidine is generic for ZANTAC and it is an H2-histamine blocker used to treat ulcers, GERD, and other gastric hypersecretory conditions.

30.

D. LASIX is a brand name for furosemide. Bumetanide is generic for BUMEX, amiloride is generic for MIDAMOR, and spironolactone is generic for ALDACTONE.

31.

A. Ethinyl estradiol/norethindrone is a combination found in oral contraceptives and, therefore, used for the prevention of pregnancy.

32.

C. Clonazepam can be dosed as 1.5 mg/day in three divided doses.

33.

D. Pravastatin is generic for PRAVACHOL. PROCARDIA is the brand name for nifedipine, PRECOSE is the brand name for acarbose, and PRONESTYL is the brand name for procainamide.

34.

D. PLAQUENIL is the brand name for hydroxychloroquine. Hydroxocobalamin is generic for VI-TAMIN B_{12}, plicamycin is generic for MITHRACIN, and hydroxyprogesterone is generic for HYLUTIN.

35.

C. PLAVIX is given 75 mg once a day. It can be given in as a loading dose of 300 mg at once if needed.

36.

A. Clonazepam is a benzodiazepine. As with all benzodiazepines, one of the most common side effects is drowsiness.

37.

B. PROZAC is the brand name for fluoxetine. Fluconazole is generic for DIFLUCAN, fluphenazine is generic for PROLIXIN, and flurazepam is generic for DALMANE.

38.

B. TAXOL is generic for paclitaxel. Pamidronate is generic for AREDIA, pancrelipase is generic for PANCREASE, and tamoxifen is generic for NOLVADEX.

39.

B. The sustained-release form of nifedipine should not be chewed or opened because it would destroy the integrity of tablet formulation and its pharmokinetic properties.

40.

C. Glipizide and NSAIDs are highly protein bound and this could lead to an increase in blood concentration of either glipizide or NSAIDs.

41.

B. Glipizide is generic for GLUCOTROL. DIABETA is a brand name for glyburide, ORINASE is a brand name for tolbutamide, and TOLINASE is a brand name for tolazamide.

42.

C. Penicillin VK has the commonly reported side effect of diarrhea.

43.

B. Simvastatin is in the HMG-CoA reductase group, which is a group of anithyperlipidemic drugs.

44.

A. Diphenhydramine is used for allergies and works as an H1-antagonist. Omeprazole is used for hypersecretory disorders and is a proton pump inhibitor, while cimetidine and nizatidine are also used for hypersecretory disorders but are H2-antagonists.

45.

B. DIFLUCAN is the brand name for fluconazole. Ketoconazole is generic for NIZORAL, itraconazole is generic for SPORANOX, and miconazole is generic for MICATIN.

46.

B. Benzodiazepines normally end with "azepam" in their names. These include lorazepam and clonazepam. They are used to treat anxiety.

47.

D. Omeprazole is part of the proton pump inhibitors, which are used to treat ulcers and help to lower the secretion of stomach acids that cause esophagitis and GERD.

48.

B. Sertraline is ZOLOFT and is part of the SSRI family of antidepressants.

49.

C. Paclitaxel is dosed 135–175 mg/m^2 and given over 3 hours every 3 weeks for breast or ovarian carcinoma.

50.

B. Since penicillin VK is an antibiotic, it is very important for the patient to finish all medication unless otherwise directed by the physician in order to thoroughly kill the bacteria and not create any bacteria, the so-called "superbug," that could be become resistant to penicillin.

51.

C. Hydroxychloroquine is known to cause gastrointestinal disturbances.

52.

A. Methotrexate is usually taken on an empty stomach.

53.

D. Simvastatin is a HMG-CoA reductase inhibitor and it is known to cause cramps, constipation, and headache.

54.

C. Amoxicillin is an antibiotic, and as with all antibiotics, it will change the content of bacteria in the stomach; oral contraceptives need specific bacteria in order to be activated.

55.

C. ANAPROX is a brand name for the generic drug, naproxen. Nalaxone is generic for NARCAN, amrinone is generic for INOCOR, and nandrolone is generic for DURABOLIN.

56.

B. Ethinyl estradiol/levonorgestrel is an oral contraceptive and it has the possibility of causing fetal damage; however, there is no definitive evidence of this occuring.

57.

B. Phenazopyridine is the drug used for urinary pain and discomfort. Even though ibuprofen is used for pain, it is not indicated for urinary pain.

58.

D. Lovastatin, gemfibrozil, and nicotinic acid are all antihyperlipidemic agents and are used to lower lipid levels. Nystatin is an antifungal.

59.

A. Warfarin can cause discoloration of urine or feces due to the metabolites of the drug.

60.

D. Lisinopril is generic for both ZESTRIL and PRINIVIL. DIURIL is the brand name for chlorothiazide.

61.

D. CECLOR is the brand name for cefaclor. Cephalexin is generic for KEFLEX, cephradine is generic for VELOSEF, and cefuroxime is generic for both ZINACEF and CEFTIN.

62.

B. Cyclophosphamide is a generic name for CYTOXAN. CYLERT is the brand name for pemoline.

63.

C. PEPCID is the brand name for famotidine. Ranitidine is generic for ZANTAC, cimetidine is generic for TAGAMET, and nizatidine is generic for AXID.

64.

D. Ciprofloxacin should not be given with dairy products due to possible binding with calcium and leading to lower concentration of ciprofloxacin in the blood.

65.

C. Tetracycline has bacteriostatic effects that could inhibit the bactericidal effects of penicillin VK.

66.

D. Cimetidine decreases the metabolism of warfarin and theophylline, leading to a decrease in elimination of the two drugs and an increase in serum concentration that could lead to warfarin or theophylline toxicity.

67.

B. NORVASC is indicated for hypertension.

68.

D. Choices A–C are all possible frequency and amounts that phenytoin can be given. The choice of which frequency and quantity depends on serum concentrations and the severity of the seizures for the specific patient.

69.

B. Diclofenac is an NSAID. NSAIDs are known to cause gastrointestinal problems and disturbances due to their activity on the intestinal lining and mucosa.

70.

B. TRIPHASIL 28 is the brand name for ethinyl estradiol/levonorgestrel. Ethinyl estradiol is just an estrogen used in combination with a progestin, conjugated estrogens are generic for PREMARIN, and ethinyl estradiol/norethindrone is generic for a variety of brand-name oral contraceptives.

71.

D. Barbiturates lead to an increase in activity of liver enzymes and this leads to greater metabolism of warfarin and less anticoagulant effect. H2-antagonists and sulfa antibiotics are the opposite. They decrease liver enzyme activity and lead to an increase in warfarin effects.

72.

D. All of the above questions would be appropriate to ask a patient regarding BACTRIM. It is important to determine the knowledge of the patient regarding their therapy and since BACTRIM contains sulfa, asking about allergies is important.

73.

D. Cephalosporins, penicillins, and erythromycin have activity against gram-positive organisms, while metronidazole has activity against the mycobacterium.

74.

C. Furosemide leads to hypokalemia. Hypokalemia is believed to lead to a reduction in activity of hypoglycemic agents.

75.

B. Diphenylhydantoin is a phenytoin and is used for seizures. The other medications are all for seasonal allergies.

76.

D. Loratidine is generic for CLARITIN. CLAFORAN is the brand name for cefotaxime, CLEOCIN is the brand name for clindamycin, and LOPID is the brand name for gemfibrozil.

77.

A. VASOTEC is the brand name for enalapril. Verapamil is generic for VERELAN, CALAN, and ISOPTIN, lisinopril is generic for ZESTRIL and PRINIVIL, and amlodipine is generic for NORVASC.

78.

C. Prazosin is generic for MINIPRES, MINOCIN is the brand name for minocycline, PRILOSEC is the brand name for omeprazole, and MONOPRIL is the brand name for fosinonpril.

79.

C. Insulin is used for insulin-dependent diabetes mellitus.

80.

B. Amiodarone is a generic name for CORDARONE. ADENOCARD is the brand name for adenosine, NORVASC is the brand name for amlodipine, and CORGARD is the brand name for nadolol.

81.

D. RELAFEN is the brand name for nabumetone. Ranitidine is generic for ZANTAC, nadolol is generic for CORGARD, and rifampin is generic for RIFAMATE.

82.

B. Oxaprozin is a generic name for DAYPRO, which is an NSAID.

83.

D. Cefepime is generic for MAXIPIME. It is part of the new fourth-generation of cephalosporins.

84.

B. Colchicine is given as a max of 8 mg per course of therapy.

85.

D. ZOFRAN is the brand name for ondansetron. Zolpidem is generic for AMBIEN, ofloxacin is generic for FLOXIN, and omeprazole is generic for PRILOSEC.

86.

C. Oxycodone is a narcotic medication and, being a derivative of codeine, can lead to drowsiness.

87.

C. DYAZIDE is the brand name for triamterene/hydrochlorothiazide. Triamterene is generic for DYRENIUM, chlorothiazide is generic for DIURIL, and bumetanide is generic for BUMEX.

88.

D. Loratidine, or CLARITIN, should be taken on an empty stomach. Food delays peak activity by 1 hour.

89.

D. Ciprofloxacin is a fluoroquinolone drug. As with all fluoroquinolones, the absorption of ciprofloxacin would be decreased with concomitant administration of antacids, multivitamins, and iron tablets. As for caffeine, the elimination of caffeine would decrease, leading to prolonged effects of caffeine on the body.

90.

B. Eptifibatide is an antiplatelet medication.

91.

D. Hyperglycemic agents can cause increased thirst, visual disturbances, and/or excessive urination.

92.

C. Hydroxychloroquine is a generic name for PLAQUENIL. HYDREA is the brand name for hydroxyurea, PLACIDYL is the brand name for ethchlorvynol, and PLENDIL is the brand name for felodipine.

93.

D. VOLTAREN is the brand name for diclofenac. Dicloxacillin is generic for DYNAPEN, dicyclomine is generic for BENTYL, and verapamil is generic for CALAN, ISOPTIN, or VERELAN.

94.

D. Penicillamine is a chelating agent used for heavy metal toxicity.

95.

D. Ketorolac is an NSAID and is used for short-term pain management.

96.

C. COREG is the brand name for carvedilol. Atenolol is generic for TENORMIN, esmolol is generic for BREVIBLOC, and carteolol is generic for CARTROL.

97.

A. MAXALT is indicated for migraine headaches. It is similar to IMITREX and the two drugs are in the class of 5-HT1 receptor antagonist.

98.

A. Medroxyprogesterone is a hormone, specifically a progestogen.

99.

B. BIAXIN is the brand name for clarithromycin. Erythromycin is generic for EES, ERYTHROCIN, ERYC, and E-MYCIN; streptomycin is a generic with no brand name; and vancomycin is generic for VANCOCIN.

100.

D. AVAPRO, the brand name for irbesartan, is used for hypertension; it is an angiotensin II antagonist.

101.

D. Pramipexole is indicated for Parkinson's disease. The trade name is MIRAPEX.

102.

A. ZAROXYLYN is usually dosed at 2.5–5 mg for hypertension.

103.

D. Since glyburide is given for diabetes, it is important for these patients to maintain good foot care, take care of cuts and bruises, and not to skip any meals.

104.

D. FOSAMAX is used for both Paget's disease and osteoporosis, both diseases of the bone.

105.

D. CLARITIN is a nonsedating antihistimine that can cause dry mouth as a side effect.

106.

D. Captopril is a generic name for CAPOTEN. VASOTEC is the brand name for enalapril, MONOPRIL is the brand name for fosinopril, and LOTENSIN is the brand name for benazapril.

107.

B. Dopamine is the only drug on the list that does not come as a transdermal patch; it only comes in an injectable form.

108.

C. Furosemide is a diuretic and does not have a direct relationship to insulin as the other three drugs.

109.

D. Paroxitine is PAXIL and the usual dose is 20 mg per day, with a maximum of 50 mg a day.

110.

A. Furosemide is a generic name for LASIX. LANOXIN is the brand name for digoxin, LARO-DOPA is the brand name for levodopa/carbidopa, and FORTAZ is the brand name for ceftazidime.

111.

B. Triamterene/hydrochlorothiazide is a diuretic and should be taken early in the day in order to avoid the inconvenience of nighttime trips to the bathroom.

112.

A. KLONOPIN is the brand name for clonazepam. Clorazepate is generic for TRANXENE, clonidine is generic for CATAPRES, and clozapine is generic for CLOZARIL.

113.

A. Hydroxychloroquine is an antimalarial drug.

114.

B. Paclitaxel is a generic name for TAXOL. PAXIL is the brand name for paroxetine, TALWIN is the brand name for pentazocine, and PARLODEL is the brand name for bromocriptine.

115.

B. GLUCOGPHAGE is the brand name for metformin. Glyburide is generic for MICRONASE, glipizide is generic for GLUCOTROL, and methylergononvine is generic for METHERGINE.

116.

C. ZANAFLEX is classified as a muscle relaxant used for muscle spasicity. The generic name is tizanidine.

117.

C. Medroxyprogesterone is a generic name for PROVERA. OGEN is the brand name for estropripate, MICRONOR is the brand name for norethindrone, and OVRETTE is the brand name for norgestrel.

118.

C. Celecoxib is a cox-2 inhibitor used for osteoarthritis or rheumatoid arthritis. The other three drugs are for the lowering of cholesterol through different means.

119.

D. Diclofenac is an NSAID; therefore, the patient should take it with food or milk and due to the possibility of GI bleeding, observe and report any signs of blood in stools. Due to the formulation of the tablet, it should not be crushed.

120.

D. The maximum dose for ibuprofen is 3.2 grams per day. Choice A is correct in strength but the frequency is wrong, choice B is not clear on which strength tablet it is referring to, and choice C has the wrong frequency but the right strength.

121.

D. NEO-SYNEPHRINE is the brand name for phenylephrine. Dopamine is generic for INTROPIN, pseudoephedrine is generic for SUDAFED, and norepinephrine is generic for LEVOPHED.

122.

B. Bupropion is used as an aid in smoking cessation and is also indicated for depression.

123.

B. Medroxyprogesterone, as with most hormonal supplements, can increase the body's sensitivity to sunlight. The tablet can be crushed and should not be taken on an empty stomach. It does not usually cause drowsiness.

124.

A. Naphazoline is used as a topical ocular vasoconstrictor. It is contraindicated in narrow-angle glaucoma. The other three agents are all used for the treatment of glaucoma.

125.

A. Propoxyphene napsylate/acetaminophen is a generic name for DARVOCET-N. DARVON-N is the brand name for propoxyphene napsylate alone, DARVON COMPOUND is the brand name for propoxyphene/aspirin/caffeine, and DECADRON is the brand name for dexamethasone.

126.

C. ULTRAM is classified as a non-narcotic analgesic. The other three are all considered narcotic analgesics and are controlled drugs, whereas ULTRAM is not a controlled drug. The generic name is tramadol.

127.

B. Phytanodione, or vitamin K, is used to oppose the effects of coumadin's anticlotting actions.

128.

C. ZYPREXA is classified as an antipsychotic medication.

129.

A. Glipizide is believed to increase the risk of cardiovascular mortality. This is based on studies done

with other oral sulfonylurea agents and the exact cause is still under debate.

130.

D. SINGULAIR is intended for long-term therapy of asthma and not intended for acute attacks or for emergency treatment of an asthma attack.

131.

D. Amphoterecin B is a generic name for ABELCET. NIZORAL is the brand name for ketoconazole, SPORANOX is the brand name for itraconazole, and LOTRIMIN is the brand name for clotrimazole.

132.

A. SEROQUEL is the brand name for quetiapine. Orphenadrine is generic for NORFLEX, olanzepine is generic for ZYREXA, and citolopram is generic for CELEXA.

133.

B. CIPRO is the brand name for ciprofloxacin. Ofloxacin is generic for FLOXIN, lomefloxacin is generic for MAXAQUIN, and norfloxacin is generic for NOROXIN.

134.

B. Estrogens are substances that can increase a patient's sensitivity to sunlight.

135.

C. Doxycycline does not require refrigeration. It does, however, need to be protected from light.

136.

D. Cefazolin is only available as an IV/injectable form. Cephalexin is available only as an oral form, while vancomycin and metoclopramide are available in both forms.

137.

C. The answer is arrived at by understanding that BENADRYL is an antihistamine and BENTYL is used as an antispasmodic.

138.

B. Diltiazem is a calcium channel blocking agent used for hypertension as well as angina.

139.

D. For ciprofloxacin, all of the above choices are correct. Since it is an antibiotic, the dose is determined by severity and type of infection. It is usually given q12h, though a once daily dose is sometimes given depending on the patient's age and renal function. The dosages do range from 500–1500 mg.

140.

D. Since cyclophosphamide is an antineoplastic agent, hair loss is a commonly reported side effect.

141.

C. Calcium channel products may lead to a decrease in the serum concentration of quinidine products.

142.

A. CYTOTEC should never be used in pregnant women or those who are planning to become pregnant.

143.

B. PROTONIX is the only proton pump inhibitor available in an IV form. All the others are only available in an oral form as of the writing of this book.

144.

D. Naproxen is an NSAID. It can be used for rheumatoid arthritis, dysmenorrhea, and inflammatory disease.

145.

B. Aspirin is not contained within FIORICET. FIORINAL, a controlled drug, contains aspirin.

146.

C. Ibuprofen is a generic name for MOTRIN. ORUDIS is the brand name for ketoprofen, RELAFEN is the brand name for nabumetone, and DAYPRO is the brand name for oxaprozin.

147.

A. Phenelzine and tranylcypromine are both members of a class of antidepressants called MAO inhibitors.

148.

D. Verapamil is an antihypertensive in the class of calcium channel blockers. A person taking verapamil should limit caffeine because it can increase caffeine levels. Since it is for hypertension, it is important that the patient maintain a low-sodium diet and find ways in dealing with stress in order to better control their hypertension.

149.

C. ALDACTONE is a diurectic and therefore does not have the effect of increasing fluids within the body. The other three are used to increase fluids to treat hypotensive episodes or in emergent situations.

150.

D. ARICEPT is usually given 5–10 mg at bedtime. It is a routine medication, not for prn use.

151.

B. In order to answer the question, it is important to realize that ELAVIL is the brand name for amitriptyline. MELLARIL is the brand name for thioridazine.

152.

D. Dilitiazem has an upper limit in dosing of 360 mg per day. The largest strength capsule it comes as is a 360 mg CD capsule.

153.

A. This is not a true contraindication as much as it is a therapeutic warning. If a patient is on clonidine and a beta-blocker and clonidine is intended to be discontinued in the future, then the beta-blocker should be stopped several days before clonidine is discontinued in order to avoid rebound hypertension. If a patient is to be on both, then the health care provider should be aware of this fact.

154.

B. Enoxaparin is a generic name for LOVENOX. NORMIFLO is the brand name for ardeparin, FRAGMIN is the brand name for dalteparin, and COUMADIN is the brand name for warfarin.

155.

A. MACRODANTIN is the one in the list used to treat UTI. The other three have no effect on UTI and are given for more systemic infections.

156.

B. Thalidomide is the drug used for leprosy that caused numerous birth defects before it was taken off the market. It is now back on the market and being studied for other uses besides leprosy treatment.

157.

C. Verapamil is a generic name for VERELAN. PROCARDIA is the brand name for nifedipine and NIMOTOP is the brand name for nimodipine.

158.

A. Once again, the relationship is based on identifying the brand and generic names. INDOCIN is the brand name for indomethacin and MINOCIN is the brand name for minocycline.

159.

C. All three drugs are antidepressants found in the class called SSRI, selective serotonin reuptake inhibitors.

160.

A. Ketorolac is an NSAID and can cause GI bleeding. The limit of 5 days is usually on the IV/IM form of the drug. Doubling the dose of the drug is not recommended for more pain relief; instead a different class of pain relievers should added. Of course, adding aspirin can aggravate or increase the risk of bleeding. Aspirin should be avoided with NSAID therapy.

161.

C. ALLEGRA-D contains an antihistimine and decongestant only. ENTEX contains a decongestant but also an antitussive, HUMIBID-DM contains only two antitussive ingredients, and PHENERGAN VC WITH CODEINE contains a decongestant, antitussive, and antihistimine.

162.

D. Filgrastim is a generic name for NEUPOGEN. EPOGEN and PROCRIT are brand names for epoetin alfa and NEUMEGA is the brand name for oprelvekin.

163.

C. Idoxuridine has nothing to do with the thyroid gland, it is HERPLEX and is used for viral infections. Levothyroxine is a supplement for low thyroid function, iodine is also used for diseases of the thyroid, and goiter refers to enlargement of the thyroid.

164.

A. MEVACOR is the brand name for lovastatin. Pravastatin is generic for PRAVACHOL, simvastatin is generic for ZOCOR, and gemfibrozil is generic for LOPID.

165.

D. ACE inhibitors can increase serum potassium levels. If used with potassium products or potassium-sparing diuretics, this could lead to hyperkalemia, or elevated potassium levels. High potassium levels are known to cause heart attacks and cardiac arrests.

166.

D. PHOSLO is the brand name for calcium acetate. Calcium carbonate is generic for OS-CAL and the other two are usually only found as the generic names.

167.

A. Captopril is an ACE inhibitor used for hypertension.

168.

D. Verapamil is classified as a calcium channel blocker and is used for hypertension.

169.

C. Loratidine is used to relieve symptoms of seasonal allergies; it is a nonsedating antihistamine.

170.

A. GLUCOPHAGE is started off at 500 mg qd-bid and can be increased to a maximum of 2550 mg/day.

171.

D. All three drugs are clearly "azoles" and being so, they are also antifungals. All three are not recommended to be given with phenytoin because they can raise serum phenytoin levels and cause phenytoin toxicity.

172.

C. Methylphenidate is used for attention deficit disorder, even though the actual diagnose of ADD is difficult and it's debatable whether the drug is truly needed for the condition.

173.

A. Diclofenac is an NSAID and as with all NSAIDs it has unwanted effects on gastric lining.

174.

D. ZAROXYLYN is a thiazide-diuretic. ZEBETA belongs in the class of beta-blockers.

175.

B. MUCOMYST is the brand name for acetylcysteine. Acetylcholine is generic for MICHOL-E, acetazolamide is generic for DIAMOX, and abciximab is generic for REOPRO.

176.

A. NEOSPORIN is an antibiotic drug combination that has all the ingredients listed except trimethoprim, which is part of the antibiotic drug BACTRIM.

177.

D. Amiodarone may lead to increased levels of digoxin in the blood and possible digoxin toxicity.

178.

D. Ibuprofen, naproxen, and aspirin can all cause ulceration due to the effects on the gastric lining and mucosa. Loperamide is for treatment for diarrhea and does not cause or cure ulcers.

179.

B. ACYCLOVIR is the brand name for zovirax. ZOCOR is the brand name for simvastatin, ZOLOFT is the brand name for sertraline and ZANTAC is the brand name for ranitidine.

180.

B. Since verapamil is used to lower blood pressure, patients can get lightheadedness from it.

181.

B. Phenytoin is an antiseizure medication and is part of the hydantoins class due to its chemical structure.

182.

A. Amoxicillin is an antibiotic and should be given for those infections where the causative pathogen is shown to be sensitive to it.

183.

A. Ondansetron is classified as an antiemetic medication.

184.

A. Enalapril is usually given once a day and the dose range is from 10 to 40 mg a day.

185.

D. Warfarin is used to prevent blood clotting. Therefore, it is possible to have black stools due to some bleeding, which should be reported. The use of a soft toothbrush is to prevent gum bleeding. The medication is sensitive to light and should be protected from it.

186.

A. Flushing is the most common side effect reported with nifedipine.

187.

C. SURFAK is used as a laxative while NEURONTIN is used to control seizures.

188.

B. NSAIDs can reduce the hypotensive effects of potassium-wasting diuretics.

189.

A. CARDURA is the only drug in the list that is not indicated for bladder spasms. CARDURA is indicated for hypertension and benign prostatic hyperplasia.

190.

A. Edema means an excess buildup of water in the body. Furosemide, spironolactone, and chloro-

thiazide are all diuretics used to relieve this condition. Nandrolone is an anabolic steroid used to treat breast cancer.

191.

C. SYMMETREL is not indicated to treat nausea and vomiting. It is used for either influenza A virus infection or to control Parkinson's disease.

192.

B. THORAZINE is chlorpromazine and used for controlling and treating nausea and vomiting.

193.

D. Etodolac is LODINE and is in the class of NSAIDs but is not currently available as an OTC product. All of the others are available OTC but at a lower strength than the prescription forms.

194.

D. ACE inhibitors and potassium products can lead to hyperkalemia, or high levels of potassium in the body, with the use of potassium-sparing diuretics. This could lead to fatal cardiac arrests.

195.

B. DIOVAN is the brand name for valsartan. Losartan is generic for COZAAR, irbsartan is generic for AVAPRO, and candesartan is generic for ATACAND.

196.

B. Cefprozil is an antibiotic with bactericidal activity.

197.

A. Omeprazole should not be given more than 360 mg per day depending on the condition. If high doses are necessary, it is usually given in 2–3 divided doses per day.

198.

D. Sertraline is generic for ZOLOFT. ZOCOR is the brand name for simvastatin, ZANTAC is the brand name for ranitidine, and SERZONE is the brand name for nefazodone.

199.

C. Enalapril is an ACE inhibitor and this class causes coughing.

200.

C. NSAIDs should not be given with anticoagulants because both can cause bleeding.

201.

C. Loperamide is IMODIUM and is indicated for treatment of diarrhea. Ondansetron is for nausea and vomiting, diphenhydramine is for treating allergies, and guaifenesin is for coughing.

202.

A. Clarithromycin and all macrolides should not be used with nonsedating antihistamines because the combination could cause cardiac arrhythmias.

203.

C. Desipramine is an antidepressant but does not belong in the class of SSRI like the other drugs listed.

204.

B. Warfarin is classified as an anticoagulant, a drug that prevents blood from clotting.

205.

C. Phenylbutazone is known to increase the effectiveness of oral antidiabetic medications through the competition for protein-binding sites or for urinary excretion. This may increase the likelihood of a hypoglycemic event if a patient is on an oral antidiabetic drug.

206.

B. TRICOR is used to control high cholesterol. The drug in the list that is used to control seizures is CEREBYX, a derivative of DILANTIN.

207.

C. Clonidine patches are made to be replaced every week, as nitroglycerin patches are for once a day changes.

208.

D. SLOW-K is only available currently in 8 mEq. Other potassium products are available in the other strengths listed.

209.

A. Betamethasone is the most potent ingredient in the list, while hydrocortisone and desonide are the weakest and mometasone is somewhere in the middle.

210.

C. Warfarin is used in treating blood clots.

211.

D. Quinolone antibiotics can lead to an increase in theophylline levels due to inhibition of liver enzymes; this can lead to theophylline toxicity if not monitored adequately.

212.

C. The 12.5 mg in the strength correlates to the drug hydrochlorothiazide, while the 25 correlates to losartan. HYZAAR is a combination antihypertensive medication.

213.

B. Verapamil is the generic name for ISOPTIN. PLENDIL is the brand name for felodipine, DYNACIRC is the brand name for israldipine, and CARDENE is the brand name for nicardipine.

214.

B. BREATHAIRE and BRETHINE are both brand names for terbutaline.

215.

D. Famotidine has been reported to cause all three reactions, with headache being reported most.

216.

D. LEVAQUIN is an antibiotic that is given either in IV or PO form at a usual adult dose of 500 mg.

217.

B. The 50 mg qd is the usual standard starting dose in adults for ZOLOFT. Therefore, in PROZAC's case, the starting dose is 20 mg qd.

218.

B. Hair loss has been reported (1–10%) with the use of warfarin.

219.

D. Paroxetine is an antidepressant that can cause drowsiness. Since it can cause drowsiness, the use of alcohol should be avoided.

220.

C. ROGAINE, the drug to treat thinning hair, also contains the ingredient minoxidil. First marketed as an antihypertensive, minoxidil gave the side effect of increased hair growth.

221.

B. Metronidazole is used for anaerobic infections. The other three drugs are specifically for use in fungal infections.

222.

A. Famotidine is a generic name for PEPCID. PROPULSID is the brand name for cisapride, PRILOSEC is the brand name for omeprazole, and AXID is the brand name for nizatidine.

223.

B. SSRI should never be used in conjunction with MAO inhibitors. The combination of the two types of antidepressants can lead to a fatal reaction.

224.

D. GLUCOTROL is brand name for glipizide. Glyburide is generic for MICRONASE and DIABETA, tolbutamide is generic for ORINASE, and glucagon is generic for GLUCAGEN.

225.

D. Quinidine and carbamazapine levels are increased if used with verapamil. Verapamil's metabolism is inhibited if used with cimetidine.

226.

D. Azathioprine is an immunosuppressive agent used in organ transplantation cases to prevent organ rejection.

227.

D. Ondansetron is indicated for prevention, not treatment, of nausea and vomiting, usually reserved for use with antineoplastic agents. It should be given before the chemotherapeutic agent and the max dose is 8 mg per day.

228.

C. Nifedipine is usually used for hypertension; however, it is also indicated for anginas.

229.

A. Cyclosporine concentration may be decreased due to hydantoins' ability to increase the metabolic enzymes of the liver, which lead to an increase in the metabolism and clearance of cyclosporine.

230.

A. Digoxin can lead to a loss of appetite.

231.

B. Nafcillin is an antibiotic that is given in a dose range of 1–2 gm IV q4h in patients with normal kidney function.

232.

A. Naproxen is an NSAID and with all medications in that class it can cause GI bleeding. It is recommended that NSAIDs be used for short-term treatment of pain and getting approval from a physician for longer periods of use. Discontinue use if blackened stools occur.

233.

B. Captopril is an ACE inhibitor for use in hypertension. It has been shown that NSAIDs decrease the effectiveness of ACE inhibitors.

234.

D. Epinephrine is the first-line drug used in all cardiac arrest or code blue situations in institutions.

235.

D. Macrolide antibiotics and propoxyphene analgesics inhibit the activity of the enzymes that break down carbamazepines in the liver. This could lead to increased levels of carbamazepine in the blood and possible toxicity.

236.

B. MAO inhibitors given concurrently with SSRIs lead to hypertension and serotonin syndrome.

237.

D. Insulin is the generic name for HUMULIN. DIA-BETA and MICRONASE are brand names for glipizide and GLUCOTROL is the brand name for metformin.

238.

B. Diclofenac is an NSAID and as with all medications in this class, it should be taken with food or milk.

239.

B. DILANTIN is the brand name for phenytoin. Primidone is generic for MYSOLINE, valproic acid is generic for DEPAKOTE, and mephenytoin is generic for MESANTOIN.

240.

A. Amphoterecin B can lead to nephrotoxicity; therefore, it could increase the problems of nephrotoxicity seen with gentamicin if the two drugs are given concomitantly.

241.

C. Anticoagulants, like warfarin, can lead to P-T prolongation if given with metronidazole due to increase in metronidazole toxicity.

242.

C. The primary purpose and use of digoxin is for congestive heart failure.

243.

D. CORVERT is used to terminate acute episodes of a-fib or a-flutter.

244.

D. Sertraline, paroxetine, and fluoxetine are all SSRIs, which inhibit the reuptake of serotonin, a neurotransmitter, into the cells. Cephradine is an antibiotic that does not have anything to do with neurotransmitters.

245.

A. Even though each listed is used for control of allergic conditions, CLARITIN is the only oral form and the other three are all nasal spray forms.

246.

B. Since levothyroxine is for chronic management of hypothyroidism, it is important for the patient to remember to take each dose. In addition, discontinuation of medication without approval of a physician could be detrimental to the patient due to the chronic and long-term nature of the disease.

247.

B. Co-trimoxazole would inhibit the metabolism of anticoagulants, like warfarin. This would lead to higher blood levels of warfarin and increase anticoagulant activity.

248.

B. Nefazodone can increase serum levels of clonazepam and other benzodiazepines through inhibition of metabolism. This would lead to increased levels and activities of benzodiazepines.

249.

C. PUD stands for peptic ulcer disease. Metronidazole is not indicated for treatment of hyperactive gastric acid secretion. Nizatidine and famotidine are H2-antagonists and can be used for the disease, while sucralfate is also indicated for gastric ulcers.

250.

B. Latanoprost is a generic name for XALATAN. COSOPT is a generic name for dorzolamide and timolol, TRUSOPT is generic for dorzolamide, and IOPIDINE is generic for apraclonidine.

251.

C. Acetazolamide is in the class of diuretics with carbonic anhydrase inhibitor activity.

252.

B. ROBINUL is the brand name for glycopyrrolate. Glipizide is generic for DIABETA, glyburide is generic for GLUCOTROL, and griseofulvin is generic for FULVICIN.

253.

A. Macrolide antibiotics inhibit the enzymes in the liver that metabolizes drugs, including benzodiazepines. This leads to an increase in serum levels and possible toxicity.

254.

D. PERMAX is classified as an anti-Parkinson's agent.

255.

C. Conjugated estrogens are indicated for estrogen replacement for menopausal symptoms due to a decrease in estrogen levels in this condition.

256.

A. Megestrol is the generic name for MEGACE. METFORMIN is the brand name for glucophage, MINIPRES is the brand name for prazosin, and MERREM is the brand name for meropenem.

257.

A. Rash can occur in 1–10% of patients taking fluconazole.

258.

B. Ibuprofen can increase serum levels of lithium, which can lead to lithium toxicity.

259.

C. Paclitaxel is classified as an antineoplastic agent.

260.

D. Isosorbide mononitrate is the generic name for both IMDUR and ISMO. ISORDIL is the brand name for isosorbide dinitrate.

261.

D. Levothyroxine is a generic name for SYNTHROID. SYMMETREL is the brand name for amantadine, SYNALGOS-DC is the brand name for the combination of dihydrocodeine, aspirin, and caffeine, and LEVSIN is the brand name for hyoscyamine.

262.

C. Potassium chloride is a generic name for KAY CIEL. KAOPECTATE is the brand name for kaolin pectin, KLONOPIN is the brand name for clonazepam, and KEFLEX is the brand name for cephalexin.

263.

C. Cefaclor represents the class of drugs known as antibiotic-cephalosporin.

264.

D. Ketamine is used as a general anesthetic, midazolam is used as a sedative, and fentanyl as a pain controller in surgeries.

265.

C. Ondansetron is indicated for emesis associated with emetogenic chemo agents. It should be used as a preventive measure; it is not intended for nausea and vomiting due to other factors or for use when patient is currently vomiting.

266.

B. Lisinopril is usually given up to 40 mg per day. It can be started as 5–10 mg per day.

267.

D. Constipation is a side effect of nizatidine that occurs in 1–10% of patients.

268.

D. Alprazolam should not be given with alcohol, it definitely can cause dependency, and it should be discontinued gradually or withdrawn symptoms can occur.

269.

C. Conjugated estrogens should not be taken concomitantly with tamoxifen.

270.

D. Hyoscyamine comes as an immediate release SL that is given as 0.125 mg tid-qid and as a timed-release capsule given as 0.375 mg q12h.

271.

D. Prazosin is given up to a max dose of 20 mg per day.

272.

C. COLESTID is the brand name of colestipol. Therefore, colistin would be the generic equivalent to COLY-MYCIN M.

273.

C. Both valproic acid and carbamazepine can interact with lamotrigine. Valproic acid inhibits the metabolism of lamotrigine and in turn lamotrigine enhances the metabolism of valproic acid. Carbamazepine metabolite increases, resulting in toxicity due to lamotrigine.

274.

B. EMLA is the name of the product that contains both lidocaine and prilocaine. XYLOCAINE just has lidocaine, SENSORCAINE has bupivacaine, and TUCKS PADS contains witch hazel.

275.

D. Glyburide is given up to 20 mg per day and is usually started around 5 mg per day.

276.

D. Levothyroxine can cause all of the conditions listed.

277.

D. All of the conditions listed can occur with a patient taking conjugated estrogens. This is all due to the hormonal effects of estrogen on the body.

278.

A. Influenza A can be treated by giving SYMMETREL.

279.

D. Estradiol is not used as a birth control pill; it is for hormone replacement.

280.

D. Glyburide is known by all three brand names listed.

281.

C. REMERON is used to treat depression.

282.

A. CLEOCIN is the brand name for clindamycin. Therefore, CLINORIL is the brand name for sulindac.

283.

D. CELLCEPT is an immunosuppressant.

284.

B. Nizatidine is an histamine H-2 antagonist.

285.

B. Phenytoin can cause drowsiness and should be taken with food.

286.

B. Diclofenac is an NSAID used to relieve pain and inflammation.

287.

A. Digoxin is usually given up to 0.5 mg per day due to the fear of toxicity that can occur if serum levels are too high.

288.

C. Diltiazem can cause headaches in 4.5–12% of patients.

289.

B. ARTHROTEC is the brand name for the drug containing diclofenac and misoprostol. It is an NSAID used to protect the lining of the GI tract from bleeding.

290.

D. Fluoxetine and MAO inhibitors can cause a serious, life-threatening reaction known as serotonin syndrome. SSRIs and MAOIs should never be given together.

291.

D. Paroxitine takes time for any effect to occur; therefore, it may take several weeks before any effect is actually seen. That is why dose adjustments should be made every 7 days in order to allow the previous dose adjustment time to show any effect.

292.

D. Isradipine, diltiazem, and enalapril are all antihypertensive agents. Procainamide is used to treat cardiac arrythmias like atrial flutter or atrial fibrillation.

293.

C. Flumazenil is the antidote for benzodiazepine overdose. Naloxone is for narcotic overdoses, protamine is to reverse heparin, and charcoal is for various overdoses but mainly for patients who overdosed on tricyclic antidepressants.

294.

D. Tacrolimus is an immunosuppressant drug given to patients who received an organ transplant.

295.

D. Gold sodium thiomalate is used for rheumatoid arthritis.

296.

A. ZOSYN is the brand name for piperacillin and tazobactam. Ticarcillin and clavulanate is generic for TIMENTIN, ampicillin and sulbactam is generic for UNASYN, and ticarcillin alone is generic for TICAR.

297.

C. Cimetidine leads to a decrease in the elimination of phenytoin through inhibition of the cytochrome enzymes within the liver. This could lead to phenytoin toxicity.

298.

C. Only the drug nitroglycerin can be given by all four routes.

299.

A. Since naproxen is an NSAID, it is important for the patient to take it with food or milk to avoid stomach irritation and possible GI bleeding if the stomach lining is damaged.

300.

C. NSAIDs can lead to an increased level of methotrexate in the serum, which can lead to methotrexate toxicity where renal dysfunction and respiratory problems can occur.

301.

B. All of the drugs with a "pril" ending are classified in the ACE inhibitor class.

302.

A. Cromolyn sodium is generic for NASALCROM. PROVENTIL is the brand name for albuterol, BECONASE is the brand name for beclomethasone, and FLOVENT is the brand name for fluticasone.

303.

B. Diphenhydramine is an H1-antagonist used to treat allergic reactions. It does not have any effect on cardiac arrhythmias. The other three listed are indicated for arrhythmias.

304.

D. Indinavir is a protease inhibitor. Acyclovir competes with the DNA polymerase for incorporation into the DNA strand of a virus. Stavudine and zidovudine are classified as nucleoside reverse transcriptase inhibitors.

305.

A. Hydroxychloroquine is indicated mainly for treatment of malaria.

306.

A. Naproxen should only be given to a max of around 1.5 gm per day. The risk of GI bleeding prevents it from being given any more frequently.

307.

B. Orthostatic hypotension is a common side effect seen with furosemide due to its ability to lower blood pressure. This effect is seen when a patient gets up from a sitting position too quickly.

308.

D. The patient should be warned of all the above. Aspirin should be avoided since taking nizatidine infers stomach ulcers and aspirin can make them worse. Black pepper, caffeine, and harsh spices can increase the irritation on the stomach and lead to more ulcers. Alcohol should not be taken because nizatidine itself can cause drowsiness and impair coordination and alcohol can increase the drowsiness and impairment.

309.

B. Tavist-1 contains the ingredient clemestine, which is an H1-antagonist used to relieve allergic symptoms.

310.

A. Aminoglutethimide (CYTADREN) may decrease effects of medroxyprogesterone by increasing hepatic metabolism.

311.

B. Pravastatin is usually only given up to 40 mg per day, with 20 mg qd the usual starting dose.

312.

A. Metoprolol is a beta-blocker used for hypertension. The rest are all in the class of calcium channel blockers.

313.

D. Naproxen is a generic name for NAPROSYN and ANAPROX. NALFON is the brand name for fenoprofen.

314.

A. Enalapril is an ACE inhibitor. As with all medications in this class, they can cause persistent coughing due to a specific action that they have on the body.

315.

B. Furosemide is a diuretic. Diuretics are used to remove excess water from the body. Therefore, edema, a condition characterized by excess water, would be the indicated condition.

316.

B. Vecuronium belongs in the class of neuromuscular blocking agents. It is used to paralyze a patient for surgery or for a medical procedure.

317.

C. Nizatidine is dosed at up to 300 mg per day, either given all at once or divided into two daily doses. The usual starting dose is 150 mg qd.

318.

D. Metallic taste, tongue irritation, and oral ulcers are common side effects of gold sodium thiomalate, occurring in > 10% of those taking the medication.

319.

B. Nizatidine can cause drowsiness in 1–10% of patients taking the medication.

320.

C. Minocyclines should not be given with antacids because the ingredients in antacids can bind to minocycline and this would decrease its effect.

321.

B. Those drugs ending with "dipine" belong to the class of drugs called calcium channel blockers.

322.

D. Fentanyl patches should be changed every 3 days. Clonidine patches are changed once a week and ni-

---

troglycerin and nicotine patches are changed on a daily basis.

323.

B. Nifedipine is a generic name for PROCARDIA. PROCAN is the brand name for procainamide, PRINIVIL is the brand name for lisinopril, and NAVANE is the brand name for thiothixene.

324.

B. Ipecac is used to induce vomiting. Promethazine and trimethobenzamide are for treating vomiting and charcoal is used as a binding agent for TCA overdoses.

325.

A. Epsom salt contains magnesium sulfate.

326.

C. Warfarin is a generic name for COUMADIN. WYDASE is the brand name for hyalurodinase, CALAN is the brand name for verapamil, and CAPOTEN is the brand name for captopril.

327.

B. Since amlodipine is generic for NORVASC, NAVANE is the brand name for thiothixene.

328.

B. A common side effect of ibuprofen is heartburn due to the effect on the stomach lining.

329.

D. The primary indicated use for paclitaxel is for carcinoma of the ovaries and breast.

330.

A. Chloral hydrate is used as a sedative. However, it is less used these days due to drugs like RESTORIL and AMBIEN being more effective and having less "daytime sedation."

331.

D. The three classes of drugs can all lead to interactions. Macrolide antibiotics inhibit the metabolism of lovastatin, leading to myopathy and rhabdomyolosis. Cholesterol-lowering drugs such as gemfibrozil, niacin, fenofibrate, and clofibrate can also lead to myopathy and rhabdomyolosis.

332.

B. Metronidazole is an antibiotic used to treat mainly anaerobes. The others have inotropic activity on the heart, which means it helps to keep the heart beating in conditions like congestive heart failure.

333.

D. Silver sulfadiazine is a generic name for THERMAZENE and SILVADENE. BACTRIM is generic for sulfamethoxazole/trimethoprim or cotrimoxazole.

334.

C. BETADINE is the brand name for povidone-iodine. Hexachlorophene is generic for PHISOHEX and iodine does not have a brand name associated with it.

335.

B. The maximum dose for this drug is not based on the narcotic component as much as on the acetaminophen component. There are different strengths of propoxyphene, but the most common is 100 mg. If the patient is taking DARVOCET-N 100, they are getting 100 mg of propoxyphene and 650 mg of acetaminophen. Since the max dose for acetaminophen in adults is 4 grams per day, the patient can only get 6 tablets per day or up to 600 mg of the propoxyphene, which is equivalent to 3900 mg or 3.9 grams of acetaminophen per day.

336.

B. Insulin is classified as a hypoglycemic agent. It is used to lower blood sugar levels.

337.

C. Cefaclor is a cephalosporin and is used to treat infections caused by susceptible organisms.

338.

B. COMBIVENT is composed of albuterol and ipratropium. The other combinations do not exist on the market at this time.

339.

A. As with other medications used to control blood pressure, diltiazem should be discontinued on a gradual basis in order to avoid rebound hypertension. This should always be done under the supervision of a physician.

340.

B. MICRONASE is the brand name for glyburide. Glipizide is generic for GLUCOTROL, tolazamide is generic for TOLINASE, and tolbutamide is generic for ORINASE.

341.

A. Paroxetine, as with other SSRI drugs, can cause disturbances with ejaculatory activity.

342.

C. Allopurinol is a drug used to treat gout and does not have any relation to antineoplastics or chemotherapeutics.

343.

C. Diclofenac is a generic name for VOLTAREN. DIDRONEL is the brand name for etidronate, VOSOL is actually 2% acetic acid, and VIVACTIL is the brand name for protriptyline.

344.

A. LANOXIN is the brand name for digoxin. Digitoxin is generic for CRYSTODIGIN, diphenhydramine is generic for BENADRYL, and propranolol is generic for INDERAL.

345.

C. SELSUN contains the ingredient selenium sulfide. Minoxidil is the ingredient in ROGAINE.

346.

C. Diltiazem should be taken with a full glass of water to help with absorption.

347.

D. Potassium chloride should be given with labels stating the tablets should be swallowed whole and dilute before using if it is in liquid form in order to avoid having too much of the drug available to the body all at once, which could lead to cardiac problems.

348.

D. Lovastatin's usual adult dose is a max of 80 mg per day. The usual starting dose is 20 mg per day, increased gradually if needed.

349.

D. Insulin can give the side effect of metallic taste.

350.

B. CORLOPAM is indicated for severe hypertension. It is also used in patients with renal compromise because it acts on the dopamine receptors.

351.

D. Amoxicillin is generic for AMOXIL. OMNIPEN is the brand name for ampicillin, UNASYN is the brand name for ampicillin sulbacatam, and ERYTHROCIN is the brand name for erythromycin.

352.

B. LOMOTIL is a narcotic drug classified as an antidiarrheal agent.

353.

D. Patients taking phenytoin should be warned of all three. The blood levels are sensitive to changing manufacturers. The drug does cause drowsiness and it should be taken with food.

354.

A. Fluconazole is an antifungal medication. As with all anti-infectives, it is important for the patient to complete the course of therapy as prescribed. The tablet can be chewed or crushed.

355.

D. Cefaclor's dosing is usually given every 8–12 hours and adults tend to get 350–500 mg q8h. Children have a dose range of up to 40 mg/kg/day.

356.

D. Ketorolac can lead the patient to a feeling of drowsiness

357.

D. Omeprazole is for ulcers or an increase in gastric reflux or stomach acid production. Therefore, it should be taken before eating. It should not be chewed or broken open because it is a sustained release medication.

358.

D. Acetaminophen toxicity can occur if all three drugs listed are given concurrently because all inhibit the metabolism of acetaminophen, leading to buildup in the liver and possible liver damage.

359.

B. Potassium-sparing diuretics help to keep potassium in the body, so by administering them with potassium chloride, the level of potassium can increase, which would lead to cardiac failure or cardiac arrest.

360.

B. Fluconazole does not have any activity to reduce inflammation; it is an antifungal. The others do have activity to treat inflammation because all three are NSAIDs.

361.

C. Lisinopril is an ACE inhibitor usually used to control hypertension.

362.

C. Gold sodium thiomalate is a rheumatoid arthritic agent.

363.

D. Sertraline is an SSRI and can lead to sexual dysfunction. In addition, the effect of it would take weeks to manifest, so changes should not be made too rapidly. A 1-week interval between dose changes should be allowed for the body to react to the drug.

364.

A. Diltiazem is a generic name for CARDIZEM. TENORMIN is the brand name for atenolol, ISOPTIN is the brand name for verapamil, and PLENDIL is the brand name for felodipine.

365.

B. Copper sulfate is not considered an electrolyte. In parenteral nutrition, copper is usually found within the trace elements. Copper is not essential to bodily functions as are electrolytes.

366.

B. A side effect of nabumatone, being an NSAID, would normally be heartburn.

367.

D. Since glipizide is used to control sugar levels, it is important that patients do not skip meals and do not double up on doses. These two things can alter the blood sugar levels in the body.

368.

D. Corticosteroids, thyroid hormones, and oral contraceptives can all decrease the effect of insulin on the body.

369.

B. Methylprednisolone is a steroid.

370.

A. Ranitidine is the H2-antagonist listed of the four drugs.

371.

C. Furosemide is a diuretic that also leads to a decrease of potassium level in the body. The others are made to spare potassium from being eliminated from the body.

372.

D. For digoxin, visual disturbances can be induced if there is an overdose of digoxin and the amount in the blood reaches a high level. It is important to notify a physician if this happens.

373.

A. Clarithromycin dose frequency can range from BID to TID depending on the infection. The same can be said of the amount. It can range from 250–500 mg depending on the type of infection and the duration needed.

374.

D. Omeprazole is for treatment of increased stomach acid production, so there would be changes in bowel movement if the drug is given since it affects the stomach.

375.

B. The generic name for ALTACE is ramipril. Ranitidine is generic for ZANTAC, rifampin is generic for RIMACTANE, and ritodrine is generic for YUTOPAR.

376.

B. Ondansetron is generic for ZOFRAN. ZYLOPRIM is the brand name for allopurinol, ONCOVIN is the brand name for vincristine, and ZOSYN is the brand name for piperacillin/tazobactam.

377.

A. Lovastatin is for lowering of cholesterol level. The use of the medication is more effective if the patient remembers to use it in conjunction with a low-fat diet.

378.

D. Phenytoin can cause a decrease in effectiveness of ethinyl estradiol/norethindrone, while the toxicity of theophylline and metoprolol can be increased if given with the oral contraceptive.

379.

B. Piroxicam is an NSAID and is not used for the treatment of gout. The other drugs listed are for the treatment of gout.

380.

D. Enalapril is generic for VASOTEC. VASOCIDIN is the brand name for an ophthalmic product that contains sulfacetamide and Prednisolone. VASODILAN is the brand name for isoxuprine, and VASCOR is the brand name for bepridil.

381.

A. A patient taking hydroxychloroquine should be instructed to take it with food or milk. This is to prevent the possibility of an upset stomach while taking the drug.

382.

A. Glipizide is for noninsulin-dependent diabetes mellitus, also known as type II diabetes.

383.

C. DILANTIN (phenytoin) should be taken with food.

384.

B. Conjugated estrogens can be taken up to 30 mg per day in three divided doses. The high end dosing is seen in patients with breast cancer palliation and metastatic diseases in some patients.

385.

B. PRILOSEC should not be crushed or chewed and must be swallowed whole due to the sustained-release formulation of the capsules.

386.

A. ACE inhibitors and allopurinol can lead to Steven-Johnson syndrome, which is a severe allergic drug reaction characterized by blisters breaking out on the lining of the mouth, throat, anus, genital area, and eyes.

387.

B. Fluoxetine belongs in the class of SSRI antidepressants. These drugs are known to take a long period of time before any observable response can be seen.

388.

A. Doxazosin is an alpha-blocker used for hypertension and for urinary outflow obstruction.

389.

C. INTRALIPIDS are also known as fat emulsions.

390.

B. AXID is the brand name for nizatidine. Nifedipine is generic for PROCARDIA, niacin does not have any specific brand name, and azathioprine is generic for IMURAN.

391.

D. The relation in this problem is that aminophylline is classified as a bronchodilator and amitriptyline is classified as an antidepressant.

392.

A. Colchicine's primary indicated use is for the treatment of gouty arthritis.

393.

A. In this relationship, protamine is the treatment for overdosing of heparin. Therefore, the treatment for digoxin overdosing is digibind.

394.

A. Lisinopril, as in all ACE inhibitors, can give the side effect of coughing.

395.

D. Ergocalciferol is vitamin E. Another name for vitamin E is tocopherol.

396.

C. The effects of levothyroxine can take some weeks before a noticeable effect is seen. This is due to the fact that it takes time for blood levels of the drug to build up.

397.

C. Allopurinol inhibits the metabolism of azathioprine, leading to possible toxicity.

398.

C. The generic name for QUINORA is quinidine; therefore, the relationship is completed by realizing that the generic name for QUINAMM is quinine.

399.

A. Ranitidine's usual adult dose is 300 mg daily or 150 mg b.i.d.

400.

A. Candida, mumps, and tuberculin are all part of the anergy panel.

401.

B. Each institution may have its own policies on changing out of tubing for propofol, but the standard is at least every 12 hours. Since there are fats in propofol, the risks of an infection increase as the length of time the tubing is up. Therefore, the sooner it is changed, the better.

402.

A. Insulin must be refrigerated at all times and shaken before use. However, it is recommended that it should be "rolled" in the hand, not shaken, in order to avoid foaming.

403.

D. If there is clumping or frosting, then the vial or syringe should be discarded because precipitation could have built up. Exercise is always the first indication of treatment for high blood sugar and any sign of illness can change your body's requirement for insulin due to the physiological changes a body undergoes during a period of ill health.

404.

C. Digoxin's action leads to a lower level of potassium in the body due to inhibition of sodium/potassium ATPase pump. This keeps potassium in the cells. The increased level of sodium outside helps to increase contractility in the heart muscles and helps those with congestive heart failure. The orange juice and banana intake helps to keep the level of potassium in the blood at a normal level.

405.

A. Phenytoin can lead to slurred speech due in part to causing drowsiness in the patient.

406.

D. H2-antagonists are used to treat gastric ulcers, while the H1-antagonists are for allergies.

407.

B. Nizatidine is an H2-antagonist; therefore, it is used for duodenal ulcers.

408.

C. Ketoprofen is an NSAID and it can lead to indigestion due to effects on the stomach lining.

409.

B. Ketorolac can cause drowsiness or dizziness.

410.

B. Prazosin can cause drowsiness or dizziness, which is why it's advised that the daily doses are taken at bedtime.

411.

C. Diclofenac can lead to decreased effectiveness of thiazide antihypertensive drugs.

412.

B. Ranitidine is not a platelet inhibitor; it is an H2-antagonist used for gastric ulcers.

413.

D. Benzonatate is used for treatment of coughing. Bumetanide is a diuretic, benzoly peroxide is an antiseptic cleanser, and benzodiazepines is a class of drugs for anxiety.

414.

D. Ibuprofen can sometimes cause drowsiness and should be tested before taking before driving or at work. As with all NSAIDs, there is a risk of GI bleeding, so report to a doctor or pharmacist any heartburn or stomach pain that has persisted.

415.

D. Salt substitutes may contain more potassium and this could be detrimental to a patient already on potassium. Liquid, powder, and effervescent tablets must be dissolved before taking and wax coating from tablets may be eliminated intact in stools, which is normal.

416.

C. FOLEX is the brand name for folic acid. Metaproterenol is generic for ALUPENT, methotrexate is generic for RHEUMATREX, and flutamide is generic for EULEXIN.

417.

C. Digoxin is classified as a cardiovascular agent used for congestive heart failure.

418.

D. Methotrexate has been used for all of the conditions listed.

419.

D. VANTIN is a cephalosporin. Since it is an antibiotic, the patient must be reminded to take the entire course of therapy and to take it around the clock. It should be refrigerated and good for 14 days, not to be frozen.

420.

C. Pravastatin given with gemfibrozil can lead to myopathy and rhabdomyolysis.

421.

A. Dopamine is usually started out at 1–5 mcg/kg/min. The dose is increased as the condition of the patient worsens or upon the physician's discretion.

422.

C. SINEMET comes as all the strengths listed except 75/200.

423.

D. Nizatidine can decrease the absorption of itraconazole and ketoconazole if given orally.

424.

D. Metoclopramide would not need any loading dose in order to achieve a desired blood level. All of the other three would require a loading dose to get a desired level quickly.

425.

C. Clonazepam is primarily indicated for seizures. Clonazepam is a benzodiazepine, but in this case, it is a treatment for seizure instead of anxiety.

426.

C. Palcitaxel is given by the IV route.

427.

B. A common side effect of ranitidine is nausea.

428.

B. For the sustained release form of diltiazem, it should not be crushed; it must be swallowed whole.

429.

C. For digoxin, visual disturbances usually indicate a toxic level is in the body.

430.

B. The drug EULEXIN is used to treat prostate cancer. NOLVADEX is used for breast cancer. VIAGRA is for sexual disturbance and WELL-COVORIN is used with flurouracil to treat malignancy.

431.

A. Amoxicillin is classified as a beta-lactam antibiotic.

432.

B. One of the indicated uses for medroxyprogesterone is endometrial carcinoma.

433.

C. Digoxin tablets are usually given once a day. Ampicillin is given q6h. Carisoprodol is given three to four times a day. Acetaminophen can be given q4–6h depending on dose.

434.

D. For enalapril, the fetus can be harmed if the drug is given during the second and third trimesters. For the first trimester, it is suggested that the drug not be used.

435.

C. Potassium chloride is an electrolyte.

436.

D. Gastrointestinal disturbances can occur in >10% of patients who take glipizide.

437.

B. Potassium-wasting diuretics have a chance to increase the toxicity of digoxin.

438.

B. Amlodipine works by inhibiting calcium ion to enter the slow channels. This leads to dilation of coronary vessels by relaxing the smooth muscles of the coronary vessel.

439.

D. All of the strengths listed are found for insulin.

440.

D. Phenytoins are primarily given to treat seizures. Tonic-clonic is a specific type of seizure.

441.

A. Alcohol is advised to be avoided while taking sertraline, even though alcohol has been shown to increase sertraline's effect.

442.

B. Z-PACK is a package that contains a specific amount of azithromycin for the patient to take. There are six tablets and the patient must take two immediately and then take one tablet once a day for the next four days until all are taken.

443.

D. Simvastatin is an HMG-CoA reductase inhibitor. These types of drugs are for the treatment of high cholesterol levels.

444.

D. The brand names for fluticasone are FLONASE and FLOVENT. FLONASE is a nasal spray while FLOVENT is an oral spray or oral powder. BECONASE is the brand name for the nasal form of beclomethasone.

445.

B. Sertraline is usually given 50–100 mg per day up to a max of 200 mg per day.

446.

D. ZANTAC and XANAX are brand names. XANAX refers to alprazolam and ZANTAC refers to ranitidine.

447.

C. Lovastatin should be taken with the evening meal. This could be due to lovastatin having a better absorption profile with food or just to overcome possible nausea while on the drug.

448.

A. SOMA COMPOUND contains carisoprodol and aspirin. SOMA alone contains just carisoprodol. The other combinations listed are not available at the time of writing the text.

449.

B. Glyburide use can lead to gastrointestinal disturbances in >10% of patients.

450.

A. Potassium chloride could lead to unwanted flatulence in >10% of patients.

451.

C. Beta-blockers, due to their actions on the body's beta receptors, have been known to mask the signs and symptoms of diabetes or high blood sugar.

452.

B. TOPROL XL is mainly used to treat hypertension. It is an extended-release form of the drug metoprolol.

453.

C. ACTOS is the brand name for pioglitazone. Glimepiride is generic for AMARYL, acarbose is generic for PRECOSE or PRANDASE, and miglitol is generic for GLYSET.

454.

B. Omeprazole is available as a sustained-release capsule. Therefore, the patient must swallow it whole and not open it or crush it.

455.

B. Fluoxetine, an SSRI, has caused drowsiness in >10% of patients who have taken it.

456.

B. Ciprofloxacin is classified as a fluoroquinolone antibiotic. It should be used for infections caused by susceptible strains of organisms.

457.

D. The usual adult dose for ZOSYN is 3.375 gm IV q6h. The other doses can also be given but they are more for patients with an impaired renal system.

458.

A. Captopril's maximum dose is 150 mg three times a day or 450 mg in one day.

459.

C. Nisoldipine has been documented to lead to headaches in 22% of patients who took the drug.

460.

D. Hydroxychloroquine is used to treat malarial infections, among other ailments. Since it is an anti-infective, the full course of therapy should be completed. The patient does become more sensitive to sunlight while on the drug and ringing in the ear is a side effect associated with it.

461.

D. Thiazides may decrease the effectiveness of glyburide. For NSAIDs and salicylates, these drugs are highly protein bound. Glyburide is also highly protein bound. Therefore, NSAIDs and salicylates can displace glyburide from the protein and increase glyburide toxicity.

462.

A. Pravastatin is for lowering of cholesterol levels. The first treatment for high cholesterol should be diet and exercise. Pravastatin has a higher effective rate if the patient continues to watch his/her diet while on the drug.

463.

C. Conjugated estrogens have shown to be very unsafe if used during pregnancy.

464.

B. DYNACIRC is used to treat hypertension. GLUCOVANCES is used to treat diabetes.

465.

D. LUPRON, leuprolide the generic, is used to treat advanced prostate carcinoma.

466.

A. Verapamil may cause increased serum levels of prazosin and can lead to sensitivity to postural hypertension.

467.

B. PERSANTINE and PLAVIX are both classified as blood thinners or antiplatelet agents. VIOXX is for treatment of arthritis and is classified as a COX-2 inhibitor, same as CELEBREX.

468.

D. Amikacin is an anti-infective placed with the aminoglycosides.

469.

A. Warfarin can cause a change in urine color. If the urine color is red or dark brown, then the patient must contact their doctor or health professional immediately. It could be a sign of bleeding due to too high a level of the drug.

470.

D. Phenytoin and carbamazepine can lead to an increase in elimination of donezepil. Quinidine can inhibit the metabolism of donezepil.

471.

D. MINIPRESS is the brand name for prazosin. Pravastatin is generic for PRAVACHOL, minoxidil is generic for ROGAINE or LONITEN, and propofol is generic for DIPRIVAN.

472.

B. Flatus is commonly seen in 3.7–4.5% of the patients taking lovastatin.

473.

C. Amoxicillin is an antibiotic and it should be taken around the clock in equal intervals.

474.

A. Patients taking loratadine should drink fluid liberally because it can cause dry mouth.

475.

B. Pramoxine is used to cure hemorroids for mothers who just gave birth. Silver sulfadiazine is used to treat burns.

476.

B. Trizaole antifungal agents can lead to increased levels of loratadine, but no serious adverse cardiac effects are seen.

477.

A. Protease inhibitors are used to treat HIV infection.

478.

A. The usual starting dose for venlafaxine extended-release is 75 mg per day with food. In some patients, it can be started at 37.5 mg per day for a few days then increase to 75 mg.

479.

D. Potassium chloride is usually given to treat conditions of hypokalemia.

480.

C. DEMADEX and LASIX are diuretics. TRANDATE is a beta-blocker. LOPRESSOR is the only beta-blocker in the choices.

481.

C. Diltiazem is listed as a cardiovascular agent in the calcium channel blocker class.

482.

D. ROBINUL is the brand name for glycopyrrolate. Glipizide is generic for GLUCOTROL, gabapentin is generic for NEURONTIN, and gancyclovir is generic for CYTOVENE.

483.

C. Antacids can lead to a decrease in absorption of MACRODANTIN.

484.

C. TRENTAL is usually started at 400 mg tid.

485.

D. Phenytoin is a generic name for DILANTIN. VANTIN is the brand name for cefpodoxime, NEURONTIN is the brand name for gabapentin, and ZARONTIN is the brand name for ethosuximide.

486.

D. Medroxyprogesterone can cause all of those listed. It can increase the chances of bleeding and lead to edema due to the steroid characteristics of it. The changes in menstrual flow are due to the actions on the hormonal system of the body.

487.

A. Simvastatin is usually given up to 40 mg per day.

488.

A. The generic name for BETOPTIC is betaxolol. The generic name for TIMOPTIC is timolol.

489.

B. BRICANYL is used to treat asthma and to open the airway. This can lead to actions on the nervous system that could increase possibility of nervousness.

490.

A. Ciprofloxacin and other fluoroquinolones should not be taken with antacids if at all possible due to increased binding of the drug to components of antacids.

491.

C. Ranitidine can cause drowsiness in some patients who take the drug.

492.

D. Fluconazole can inhibit the metabolism of warfarin and can increase the effects of it.

493.

D. Paclitaxol should not be put in a PVC bag due to possible reaction with the plastic and the drug attaching to the bag and not actually being delivered to the patient.

494.

B. DESOWEN is the brand name for desonide. Betamethasone is generic for ULTICORT or DIPROSONE, halcinonide is generic for HALOG, and halobetasol is generic for ULTRAVATE.

495.

D. Patients taking prazosin must monitor their blood pressure since it is for lowering of blood pressure, maintain a low-sodium diet to keep blood pressure lowered, and rise slowly from a sitting or lying position since the drug can cause orthostatic hypotension if the patient stands up too fast or too suddenly.

496.

D. Ipecac syrup is used to induce vomiting. Promethazine and ondansetron are used to prevent it and bisacodyl is used to induce a bowel movement.

497.

B. NEORAL can be mixed with orange juice for better taste. NEORAL and SANDIMMUNE should never be used interchangeably. A patient should always take one or the other without switching between the two.

498.

A. Levothyroxine is given for underactive thyroid.

499.

D. Propoxyphene can inhibit the metabolism of carbamazepine and can possibly lead to toxicity of carbamazepine.

500.

C. Azelastine is the only one listed that is available as a nasal spray. The others are only available in oral dosage forms.

501.

C. Medroxyprogesterone dosing is disease state–dependent, so the doctor will make the determination on the dose for each patient based on disease state.

502.

C. ZANAFLEX is used for muscle relaxation so daytime sedation is a problem.

503.

B. K-CLOR is the brand name for potassium chloride. KLONOPIN is the brand name for clonazepam, PLENDIL is the brand name for felodipine, and PRODIUM is the brand name for phenazopyridine.

504.

A. NORFLEX is a skeletal muscle relaxant.

505.

B. NSAIDs can increase the antihypertensive actions of CARDURA.

506.

D. Diltiazem and beta-blockers could lead to increased cardiac depression. However, physicians will prescribe both to a patient if his/her blood pressure is not controlled with either one of the drugs alone.

507.

B. Penicillin G Procaine is the long-acting form and is given by the IM route.

508.

C. CORTISPORIN contains neomycin, polymixin B, and hydrocortisone. Choice A, without the hydrocortisone, is known as NEOSPORIN and choice D is known as POLY-PRED. There is no such product for choice C.

509.

D. Conjugated estrogens can lead to increased sensitivity to sunlight; therefore, it is recommended that the patient avoid prolonged exposure to sunlight.

510.

A. BENADRYL is the brand name for diphenhydramine. Dimenhydrinate is a generic for DRAMAMINE.

511.

C. Enalapril belongs to the class of drugs known as ACE inhibitors.

512.

B. Protamine is used as an antidote for heparin overdose. Digoxin immune fab is used as an antidote for digoxin overdose.

513.

D. Captopril is not advised for pregnant women in the second and third trimester. It is also recommended to be given 1 hour before meals and can be found in the milk of nursing mothers.

514.

B. The maintenance dose is between 2–10 mg qd. The therapeutic range is dependent on each patient and loading doses can vary if a physician does choose to give a loading dose.

515.

C. Mupirocin is a topical anti-infective agent. Its brand name is BACTROBAN.

516.

A. Piroxicam is used to treat inflammation. Propafenone is used to treat arrythmias.

517.

D. Nabumetone can lead to increased bleeding potential if given with warfarin.

518.

B. The brand name for clarithromycin is BIAXIN. ERYTHROCIN is the brand name for erythromycin, ZITHROMAX is the brand name for azithromycin, and CLEOCIN is the brand name for clindamycin.

519.

A. Patients taking aspirin should always be reminded to take it with food or milk.

520.

B. Due to its actions on alpha-receptors, prazosin can lead to orthostatic hypotension.

521.

D. Clarithromycin is not suggested for pregnant women if possible. The suspension is one of the few antibiotic suspensions that should not be refrigerated because it tastes better at room temperature. As with most suspensions mixed up, it is good for only 14 days.

522.

B. Flecainide is used to treat arrythmias. Clomipramine is used to treat depression.

523.

B. Captopril is used mainly to treat hypertension.

524.

D. Fluoxetine is not to be taken with alcohol and the response of the drug does take several weeks to be seen. It can cause drowsiness, so it must be taken with care.

525.

B. Lisinopril should be dispensed with the auxillary label "May cause drowsiness or dizziness."

526.

C. Since phenytoin levels must be measured, it is suggested that a patient does not change the brand that he or she takes. This could change the effects of the drug.

527.

C. Sertraline should not be taken with alcohol.

528.

A. Levothyroxine can lead to increased toxicity of anticoagulants like warfarin.

529.

B. Cefuroxime is an antibotic. All antibiotics interact with oral contraceptive drugs because oral contraceptives need the bacteria in the gut to be active and antibiotics kill those off.

530.

A. A patient should be aware that acid secretions increase at around 7 PM and taking it at 6 PM would help to reduce and alleviate it.

531.

A. Patients taking conjugated estrogens should have increased vitamin B-6 and folic acid intake.

532.

D. Smoking can lead to decreased effects of the drug. Since propoxyphene is a narcotic, it should not be taken with alcohol and other sedatives because those can potentiate the drowsiness that propoxyphene causes.

533.

B. Loratidine should be taken with plenty of water.

534.

C. Clarithromycin is given for mainly respiratory infections and to only the strains of pathogens that are susceptible to it.

535.

D. The usual adult range to start is 10–20 mg tid. However, it can be increased and patients can take the extended-release form of it qd.

536.

B. Ethinyl estradiol/levonorgestrel can lead to increased theophylline toxicity.

537.

B. Ranitidine can lead to a decreased absorption of ketaconazole.

538.

C. Azelastine is a generic name for ASTELIN.

539.

B. For famotidine, a once-daily dose should be taken at bedtime because of increased nighttime secretion of acid.

540.

C. The ketorolac brand name in the ophthalmic form is ACULAR. STADOL is the brand name for butorphanol, TORADOL is the brand name for ketorolac in the oral form, and AGGRENOX is the brand name for the combo asprin/dipyridamole.

541.

B. One of the side effects of taking aspirin is tinnitus. Tinnitus is also a sign of aspiring overdose.

542.

D. THORAZINE is the brand name for chlorpromazine. DIABINESE is the brand name for chlorpropamide.

543.

C. MEGACE is also given for appetite stimulation and for weight gain.

544.

B. Fluconazole is an antifungal; therefore, it is given for candida infections.

545.

A. Hydroxyzine is the generic name for ATARAX. ATIVAN is the brand name for lorazepam.

546.

D. Minocycline is not for women who are pregnant.

547.

B. Paclitaxel should not be used with plasticized PVC equipment.

548.

D. KAY CIEL is the brand name for potassium chloride. Sodium chloride has various other names. Potassium acetate does not have a brand name and calcium gluconate is also known as KALCINATE.

549.

D. Cephalexin would show a cross-sensitivity with penicillin due to the similar molecular chemical structure.

550.

D. The brand name for propranolol is INDERAL. IMDUR is isosorbide mononitrate, IMODIUM is loperamide, and INDERIDE is propranolol plus hydrochlorothiazide.

551.

B. RESTORIL is the brand name for temazepam. Diazepam is generic for VALIUM, alprazolam is generic for XANAX, and lorazepam is generic for ATIVAN.

552.

B. Alcohol is contraindicated in patients taking colchicines due to its metabolism through the liver.

553.

C. Clonazepam is a benzodiazepine; therefore, it is listed as a schedule C-IV.

554.

C. VOLMAX and VENTOLIN are different dosage forms of albuterol.

555.

A. Famotidine is indicated for reducing gastric acid secretion.

556.

A. Allopurinol could lead to increased levels of cyclophosphamide cytotoxic metabolites.

557.

A. Cefaclor could be given with food if reducing stomach upset is desired.

558.

B. Ketoconazole needs to have gastric acidity to be effective. Drugs like nizatidine that reduces acidity would inhibit the effects of ketoconazole and lead to treatment failure.

559.

D. Clonazepam is a benzodiazepine and is contraindicated with alcohol because alcohol can increase the likelihood of drowsiness and sedation and inhibit its metabolism in the liver.

560.

B. FERGON is the brand name for ferrous gluconate. Ferrous sulfate is FEOSOL, ferrous fumarate has various brand names, as do multivitamins and minerals.

561.

B. DIABETA is the brand name for glyburide. Metformin is generic for GLUCOPHAGE, glipizide is the brand name for GLUCOTROL, and insulin is generic for HUMULIN or NOVOLIN.

562.

D. TAPAZOLE is used to treat patients with hyperthyroidism.

563.

D. Cimetidine should be given with meals in order to be effective at the peak time of gastric acid secretion.

564.

D. Furosemide is a diuretic and should be taken early enough in the day to prevent nocturia and the patient should rise slowly from a lying or sitting position to avoid orthostatic hypotension.

565.

A. Patients taking colchicines should be advised to stop if GI symptoms occur.

566.

B. Calcium acetate, also known as PHOSLO, is given for hyperphosphatemia. The drug binds to phosphorus and is eliminated in the feces.

567.

B. The usual dose for amoxicillin in children is weight dependent, while in adults, it is usually 250–500 mg every 8 hours.

568.

A. NASALCROM is the brand name for cromolyn sodium. Albuterol is generic for VENTOLIN, fluticasone is generic for FLOVENT, and cimetidine is generic for TAGAMET.

569.

A. PEPCID is the brand name for famotidine. Lansoprazole is generic for PREVACID, metoclopramide is generic for REGLAN, and omeprazole is generic for PRILOSEC.

570.

C. NASACORT is the brand name for triamcinolone. Fluticasone is generic for FLONASE (nasal form), beclomethasone is generic for VANCENASE or BECONASE, and prednisolone is generic for PRED FORTE or PRELONE.

571.

B. FELDENE is the brand name for piroxicam. Sulindac is generic for CLINORIL, cyclobenzaprine is generic for FLEXERIL, and carisoprodol is generic for SOMA.

572.

A. CLINORIL is the brand name for sulindac.

573.

C. FLEXERIL is the brand name for cyclobenzaprine.

2 Mathematical and Pharmaceutical Calculations

chapter objectives

Students will demonstrate knowledge of:

➤ Basic mathematical operations such as ratio, proportion, and percentage

➤ Pharmaceutical calculations such as systems conversions and operational uses

---

DIRECTIONS Each of the questions or incomplete statements below is followed by suggested answers or completions. Select the **one answer** that is best in each case.

---

1. Given the fraction 1/20, describe it in a percentage notation.
   A. 20%
   B. 1/2%
   C. 100%
   D. 5%

2. Display 15% in decimal form.
   A. 1.5
   B. 0.15
   C. 15.0
   D. 0.015

3. What is the missing term in the proportion: X:1ml::200 mEq:50ml?
   A. 4 ml
   B. 4 mmol
   C. 4 mEq
   D. 4 mg

4. What is a valid fractional equivalent for 12.5%?
   A. 12.5/1000
   B. 125/1000
   C. 1.25/1000
   D. 0.125/1000

5. Add 22.8 mg. + 42.3 mg + 37.6 mg. + 8.4 mg.
   A. 11.11
   B. 1.111
   C. 111.1
   D. 1111.0

6. Show 1/2 as a percentage notation.
   A. 2%
   B. 3%
   C. 50%
   D. 1/2%

7. Multiply 500 and 5.0123.
   A. 250.615
   B. 2506.15
   C. 2560.15
   D. 2500.0

8. Which answer best describes the lowest fractional reduction for 25/100?
   A. 1/5
   B. 1/10
   C. 1/20
   D. 1/4

9. Convert 12% to a decimal.
   A. 1200
   B. 0.12
   C. 1.2
   D. 12

10. What is the lowest reduced fraction for 15%?
    A. 15/100
    B. 0.15/100
    C. 3/20
    D. none of the above

11. What is the missing term in the proportion: 2.4 mEq/7.2 mEq = 4%/X?
    A. 12%
    B. 0.12 mEq
    C. 0.12%
    D. 1.2%

12. Given the fraction 3/4, which answer best identifies its decimal equivalent?
    A. 3.4
    B. 0.75
    C. 0.7
    D. 0.25

13. Convert 12.5% to a fraction in lowest terms.
    A. 1/8
    B. 1/2
    C. 3/4
    D. 4/5

14. Convert 12.5% into decimal form.
    A. 1.25
    B. 12.5
    C. 0.125
    D. 125.0

15. Convert 1.7% to a decimal.
    A. 170
    B. 0.17
    C. 0.017
    D. 1.7

16. Given the word expression *three quarters,* how is it expressed numerically?
    A. 3/25
    B. 1/25
    C. 1/4
    D. 3/4

17. Convert 50% to a fraction in lowest terms.
    A. 1/2
    B. 1/4
    C. 1/8
    D. 3/4

18. Given the fraction 1/20, convert it to a decimal notation.
    A. 5.5
    B. 1.2
    C. 0.05
    D. 0.5

19. Which is the missing term in the equation: 400 mcg/X = 40 mcg/1 ml?
    A. 0.1 mcg
    B. 10 ml
    C. 0.1 ml
    D. 10 mcg

20. Given the fraction 2/5, convert it to a decimal notation.
    A. 0.4
    B. 0.2
    C. 0.02
    D. 0.05

21. Which is the missing term in the proportion: 2.4 mEq/5 ml = X/1 ml?
    A. 12%
    B. 0.48 ml
    C. 0.48 mg
    D. 0.48 mEq

22. Convert 12.5% into its lowest fractional form.
    A. 0.125/125
    B. 1/125
    C. 1/12/5
    D. 1/8

23. Multiply 2/3 by 4/5.
    A. 6/8
    B. 1
    C. 6/15
    D. 8/15

24. How would you express *three quarters* as a percent?
    A. 25%
    B. 3%
    C. 75%
    D. 2.5%

25. Subtract 90% from 100% and express the answer in decimal form.
    A. 0.1
    B. 1.9
    C. 1.0
    D. 1.9

26. Describe the fraction 25/100 verbally?
    A. twenty-five hundredths
    B. one-fifth
    C. twenty-five hundreds
    D. two and one-half

27. Divide 0.5 by 0.25.
    A. 2.0
    B. 0.2
    C. 20
    D. none of the above

28. Show 3/5 as a decimal.
    A. 0.06
    B. 0.6
    C. 0.16
    D. none of the above

29. Convert 1 1/2 to a decimal.
    A. 3.2
    B. 15
    C. 0.15
    D. 1.5

30. Show the fraction 1/4 as a percentage.
    A. 2.5%
    B. 25%
    C. 0.25%
    D. 14%

31. Which is the missing term in the proportion: 5000 units/1 ml = 1250 units/X ml?
    A. 0.5 ml
    B. 4 ml
    C. 0.25 ml
    D. 3/4 ml

32. Divide the following: 4/5 by 1/2
    A. 8/5
    B. 5/8
    C. 4/10
    D. 5/7

33. Convert 4/100 to a decimal.
    A. 0.4
    B. 0.04
    C. 0.004
    D. 4

34. Given the fraction 3/20, describe it in a percentage notation.
    A. 12%
    B. 15%
    C. 1.5%
    D. 0.15%

35. Which is the missing term in the proportion: 3/9 = _____/27?
    A. 9
    B. 12
    C. 14
    D. 6

36. Given the fraction 5/8, which answer best identifies its decimal equivalent?
    A. 0.625
    B. 0.25
    C. 0.4
    D. 0.0625

37. Add 0.056g + 0.0256g + 1.63g.
    A. 1711 g
    B. 171.1 mg
    C. 17.11 g
    D. 1711 mg

38. What is 20% of 250?
    A. 20
    B. 50
    C. 25
    D. 10

39. Which is the missing term in the expression: X/1 ml = 400 mcg/10 ml?
    A. 4 ml

B. 400 mg

C. 4 mcg

D. 40 mcg

40. Given the fraction 7/20, convert it to a decimal notation.

A. 0.35

B. 3.5

C. 0.035

D. 0.335

41. Divide 0.6875 by 0.8125.

A. 8.462

B. 8.4615

C. 0.8462

D. 84.6154

42. Which of the following best identifies the fractional notation for the expression one-tenth?

A. 1/100

B. 1/5

C. 110

D. 1/10

43. Subtract 12% from 87%.

A. 0.99

B. 7.5

C. 0.75

D. 0.075

44. *One hundred twenty-five thousandths* expressed as a decimal is?

A. 1.25

B. 12.5

C. 0.125

D. 125.0

45. What term is missing in the expression: 40 mEq/X = 120 mEq/30 ml?

A. 0.333 mEq

B. 10 ml

C. 160 mEq

D. 16 ml

46. Given the word expression *two-tenths,* express it as a percent.

A. 0.02%

B. 0.2%

C. 20%

D. 2%

47. Convert 1.5 to a percent.

A. 1.5%

B. 15%

C. 0.15%

D. 150%

48. Reduce the term *fifteen-hundredths* to its lowest value.

A. 15/100

B. 1/8

C. 1/7

D. 3/20

49. Convert 0.453 to a percent.

A. 45.3%

B. 0.453%

C. 4.53%

D. 453%

50. Given the fraction 8/40, which answer identifies its decimal equivalent?

A. 2.0

B. 0.02

C. 0.2

D. 20.0

51. Subtract 23.75 ml from 118 ml.

A. 294.25 ml

B. 9.425 ml

C. 20.9425 ml

D. 94.25 ml

52. Convert 4/12 into a percent.
    A. 33%
    B. 30%
    C. 3.33%
    D. 330%

53. Convert 1.05 to a percent.
    A. 10.5%
    B. 1.05%
    C. 105%
    D. 1%

54. Convert 75/100 into a percentage.
    A. 75%
    B. 7.5%
    C. 0.75%
    D. 175%

55. What is the missing term in 234 mg/117 mg = 23.4% /X?
    A. 0.117 mg
    B. 11.7 mg
    C. 11.7%
    D. 117%

56. Reduce 5/100 to its lowest fractional term.
    A. 5/10
    B. 1/20
    C. 1/2
    D. 5/20

57. Subtract 1.25 from 1.075.
    A. −0.175
    B. 0.175
    C. 1.750
    D. −1.750

58. Write the expression *one-tenth* as a decimal.
    A. 0.01
    B. 0.001
    C. 0.1
    D. 1.0

59. Add the following and express the answer in grams: 450 mg + 5 g + 3500 mg =
    A. 895 g
    B. 89.5 g
    C. 8.95 g
    D. 3955 g

60. What is 25% of 350 ml expressed in L?
    A. 87.5 L
    B. 87500 L
    C. 0.875 L
    D. 0.0875 L

61. Divide 0.6667 by 0.3333.
    A. 2.003
    B. 20.03
    C. 2000
    D. 2.0003

62. Write the expression two-tenths in it lowest fractional form.
    A. 1/5
    B. 1/50
    C. 2/100
    D. 2/1

63. Which is the missing term in the proportion: 5 mg/2 ml = 2 mg/X?
    A. 0.8 ml
    B. 8 ml
    C. 5 ml
    D. 5 mg

64. Given the fraction 15/100, which answer identifies the decimal equivalent?
    A. 1.5
    B. 0.15
    C. 15.0
    D. 0.015

65. Subtract 12 fl. oz. from 24.8 fl. oz.
    A. 36.8 fl. oz.

B. 1.28 fl. oz.

C. 128 fl. oz.

D. 12.8 fl. oz.

66. Write the answer to 1/2 of 5/10 as a percent.

A. 25%

B. 50%

C. 100%

D. 2.5%

67. Convert 1 to a percent.

A. 0.1%

B. 0.01%

C. 10%

D. 100%

68. Which of the following is greater than 30%?

A. 1/4

B. 1/10

C. 2/5

D. 0.05

69. Which is the missing term in the equation: 50 mEq/2.5 ml = X/4 ml?

A. 80 ml

B. 8.0 ml

C. 80 mEq

D. 80 mg

70. Which of the following is less than 50%?

A. 3/4

B. 0.85

C. 5/4

D. 0.07

71. Convert 1/4 to a percent.

A. 25%

B. 0.25%

C. 75%

D. 2.5%

72. Which answer best describes 0.05 in a word expression?

A. five-hundredths percent

B. one-fifth

C. five-hundredths

D. one-half

73. Add the following and express the answer in g: 187.4 mg + 13 g + 276 mg

A. 1.34634 g

B. 134.634 g

C. 13.4634 g

D. 134.4634 g

74. What is 65% in its lowest fractional form?

A. 13/100

B. 5/100

C. 1/5

D. 13/20

75. Convert 1.25% to an improper fraction.

A. 4/5

B. 125/100

C. 5/4

D. 100/125

76. Which number is the largest in value out of the following?

A. 0.55

B. 80%

C. 2/3

D. 5/8

77. Which term in the proportion 1/X = 8/16 is missing?

A. 12.8

B. 0.5

C. 1/2

D. 2

78. Write the expression *one hundred twenty-five thousandths* in its lowest form.
    A. 125/1000
    B. 25/200
    C. 1/8
    D. 5/40

79. Add the following: 1.374 + 1.246 + 247.3 + 0.11
    A. 260.030
    B. 2.603
    C. 26.03
    D. 2600.30

80. What is the decimal equivalent of 3/8?
    A. 0.0375
    B. 0.375
    C. 3.75
    D. 0.333

81. Which of the following is the smallest?
    A. 0.75
    B. 1/10
    C. 45%
    D. 0.35

82. What is the percent equivalent for the fraction 15/100?
    A. 15%
    B. 1500%
    C. 150%
    D. 0.15%

83. Add 127 ml + 12.7 ml + 1.25 ml + 1 L.
    A. 1140.95 ml.
    B. 11.4095 ml.
    C. 1.14095 L.
    D. answers A and C

84. Reduce 6/16 to the lowest fraction.
    A. 1/4
    B. 3/4

C. 1/8
D. 3/8

85. Divide 0.8333 by 0.50.
    A. 1.67
    B. 16.66
    C. 166.7
    D. 0.167

86. Which answer shows 45.5% as a valid fractional equivalent?
    A. 455/1000
    B. 45.5/100
    C. 455/100
    D. all of the above

87. Subtract 543.1 mg from 1000 mg
    A. 456.9 mg
    B. 45.69 mg
    C. 4.569 mg
    D. 456 mg

88. Which of the following is larger than 15% of 200?
    A. 15
    B. 30
    C. 45
    D. 4.5

89. Divide 0.65 by 0.450.
    A. 144
    B. 0.144
    C. 14.44
    D. 1.44

90. If X > 45% but X < 85%, which of the following can X *not be?*
    A. 50%
    B. 3/4
    C. 0.9
    D. 0.67

91. Multiply 80 by 3.012.
    A. 2409.600
    B. 24.96
    C. 240.960
    D. 2410

92. Which of the following is smaller than 60%?
    A. 9/10
    B. 2/5
    C. 1.1
    D. 0.8

93. Divide 23.75 by 10.2.
    A. 23.28
    B. 2.33
    C. 0.23
    D. 0.238

94. Multiply 0.5 by 3.5 and give the answer in percent.
    A. 1.75%
    B. 17.5%
    C. 175%
    D. 350%

95. Multiply 1355% and 450%.
    A. 60.975
    B. 60975
    C. 6.0975
    D. 0.60975

96. What is the lowest fractional reduction for the fraction 15/100?
    A. 4/20
    B. 3/20
    C. 1.5/100
    D. 15/10

97. Divide 0.45 by 0.650.
    A. 6.923

B. 0.69
C. 6.9
D. 69

98. The term *six and five-eighths* refers to which of the following?
    A. 65/8
    B. 6 5/8
    C. 5/8
    D. 8/65

99. Which is the missing term for 3 mMol/50 ml = 150 mMol/X?
    A. 2500 mMol
    B. 2500 ml
    C. 250 ml
    D. 2.5 mMol

100. What is the percent notation for the expression *twenty-five hundredths?*
    A. 2.5%
    B. 250%
    C. 25%
    D. 0.25%

101. Add 34.79502 + 24.1 + 14.1 + 10.1
    A. 83.09502
    B. 830.9502
    C. 83.095
    D. 83.0

102. If 30% of X is 105, what is X?
    A. 350
    B. 300
    C. 250
    D. 35

103. Multiply 0.001 by 2.102.
    A. 0.2102
    B. 21.02
    C. 0.002
    D. 2.0012

104. Give a fractional meaning to the word expression *five-hundredths*.
    A. 5/100
    B. 100/5
    C. 5/10 × 100
    D. 49.1

105. Add 0.3 + 0.08 + 0.006 + 0.105.
    A. 491
    B. 4.91
    C. 0.491
    D. 49.1

106. The decimal 0.05 can be described in what percent notation?
    A. 0.5%
    B. 0.55%
    C. 5%
    D. 5.5%

107. Multiply 06.01 by 10.60.
    A. 63.71
    B. 16.61
    C. 1.76
    D. 67.31

108. Multiply 0.45 by 2.5 and give the answer as a percent.
    A. 11.25%
    B. 1.125%
    C. 1125%
    D. 112.5%

109. Multiply 12.75 by 2.15.
    A. 27.41
    B. 0.593
    C. 59.30
    D. 5.93

110. Which of the following is the decimal form for the percentage 25%?
    A. 2.5
    B. 0.25
    C. 0.025
    D. 25.0

111. Multiply 0.9 by 1.10.
    A. 1
    B. 0.99
    C. 9.9
    D. 9.99

112. What is the answer for the following: (−1.5 × 3.5) + 5?
    A. 5.25
    B. −0.25
    C. 0.25
    D. 10.25

113. Divide 5.75 by 0.375.
    A. 15.333
    B. 1.533
    C. 0.153
    D. 153.3

114. Which of the following is a word translation for the decimal 0.15?
    A. fifteen-tenths
    B. fifteen-thousandths
    C. fifteen-hundredths
    D. fifteen-hundreds

115. Which is the missing term in X /100% = 25 g/50 g?
    A. 50%
    B. 0.5 g
    C. 5 ml
    D. 5%

116. What is (−15 + 20) ×−45?
    A. −225
    B. 225
    C. 1575
    D. −1575

117. Multiply 1.07 by 2.01.
    A. 2.16
    B. 0.0215
    C. 0.216
    D. 2.15

118. If 56% is less than X and 4/5 is greater than X, which choice could be X?
    A. 2/5
    B. 0.65
    C. 55%
    D. 1/5

119. Convert 11.5% to a decimal.
    A. 1.15
    B. 11.5
    C. 115
    D. 0.115

120. What is the percent equivalent for the fraction 1/10?
    A. 1%
    B. 100%
    C. 110%
    D. 10%

121. Subtract 0.36 from 0.375.
    A. 0.150
    B. 1.150
    C. 0.015
    D. 15.0

122. If W = 3/4, 7/10 > X > 50%, Y < 45%, and Z = 0.7, which of these is the largest?
    A. X
    B. Z
    C. W
    D. Y

123. Add 3/8 + 0.943 + 11.21 + 27.
    A. 3.9528
    B. 39.528

C. 395.289
D. 395.3

124. Which answer best shows the percent notation for the expression *one-quarter?*
    A. 4%
    B. 50%
    C. 25%
    D. 75%

125. Add one-half and 50%.
    A. 0.5
    B. 1
    C. 150
    D. 1 1/2

126. Identify the decimal notation for the expression *five-tenths?*
    A. 0.510
    B. 5.10
    C. 0.5
    D. 5.5

127. Add 32.75 g + 0.03629 g + 0.00944 g.
    A. 32.79573 mg
    B. 32.79573 g
    C. 327.9573 g
    D. 327957.3 Kg

128. Given the decimal 0.15, which is its fractional equivalent?
    A. 15/100
    B. 15/10
    C. 3/2
    D. 3/20

129. Convert 1/8 to a percent.
    A. 1.25%
    B. 12.5%
    C. 125%
    D. 0.125%

130. Which of the following is *two-tenths* expressed as a fraction?
    A. 1/10
    B. 5/10
    C. 210
    D. 2/10

131. Add 152.5 mg + 42.5 mg + 1 g + 0.1 g.
    A. 1295.0 mg
    B. 1.295 g
    C. 0.001295 Kg
    D. all of the above

132. What is 50% of 50%?
    A. 1%
    B. 25%
    C. 100%
    D. 0.25%

133. Supply the missing term in the proportion 40 mEq/20 ml = 2 mEq/ X.
    A. 0.5 mEq
    B. 1 mEq
    C. 1 ml
    D. 0.5 ml

134. What is the valid decimal equivalent for 125/1000?
    A. 0.125
    B. 1.25
    C. 12.5
    D. 0.0125

135. Convert 2/3 to a decimal.
    A. 0.67
    B. 6.7
    C. 0.066
    D. 0.067

136. How would you note the fractional equivalent for the decimal 0.05?
    A. 50/100

B. 5/10
C. 50/1000
D. 5/100

137. Add 27.4 ml + 135.5 ml + 0.1 ml + 1 ml.
    A. 164 ml
    B. 163.01 ml
    C. 0.164 L
    D. answers A and C

138. What is the lowest fractional reduction for the decimal 0.1?
    A. 1/10
    B. 1/100
    C. 10/50
    D. 1/1000

139. Divide 0.625 by 0.3125.
    A. 200
    B. 20
    C. 2.0
    D. 0.2

140. Add 1/4 and 5/12 and express the answer as a percent.
    A. 0.66%
    B. 6.67%
    C. 60%
    D. 67%

141. Subtract 5.5 cc from 240 cc.
    A. 23.45 cc
    B. 234.5 cc
    C. 2.345 cc
    D. 2.35 cc

142. Describe the decimal 0.2 as a word expression.
    A. two-tens
    B. two-hundredths
    C. two-hundreds
    D. two-tenths

143. Convert 80% to a fraction in its lowest terms.
    A. 1/5
    B. 1/8
    C. 3/4
    D. 4/5

144. Which of the following is the largest?
    A. 55 mg
    B. 2 kg
    C. 100 mcg
    D. 2.2 lb

145. Convert 0.125 to a percent.
    A. 0.125%
    B. 12.5%
    C. 1.25%
    D. 0.0125%

146. What is fifteen-hundredths of a grain written as a fraction?
    A. 15/100 gr
    B. 15/1000 gr
    C. 15/10 gr
    D. 15/1 mg

147. Subtract 0.75 g from 3.1 g
    A. −2.35
    B. 2.35
    C. 0.0235
    D. −0.235

148. What is the lowest reduced fraction for 0.25?
    A. 1/5
    B. 1/4
    C. 1/10
    D. 1/25

149. Convert 0.0075 to a percent.
    A. 7.5%
    B. 75%
    C. 0.75%
    D. 0.075%

150. Describe the decimal 0.75 in a percent notation.
    A. 75%
    B. 7.5%
    C. 0.75%
    D. 0.075%

151. Subtract 101.01 gr from 1010.101 gr.
    A. 0 gr
    B. 90.909 gr
    C. 909.091 gr
    D. 9.9091 gr

152. What is another way of expressing the words *five-hundredths?*
    A. 0.5
    B. 0.05
    C. 0.005
    D. 0.0005

153. Which is the missing term in the proportion: X/25 g = 4.06 mEq/0.5 g?
    A. 0.1624 ml
    B. 0.3248 mEq
    C. 203 mEq
    D. 20.3 mg

154. What is 0.1 written as a percent?
    A. 1%
    B. 10%
    C. 100%
    D. 1000%

155. Subtract 0.35 from 35.035.
    A. 346.9
    B. 34.7
    C. 3.469
    D. 34.685

156. Subtract 0.35 mg from 35.035 g.
    A. 35034.65 mg
    B. 35.03465 g
    C. 34.685 mg
    D. answers A and B

157. Multiply 3 mg by 11.123 mg.
    A. 333.69 mg
    B. 33.369 mg
    C. 33.639 g
    D. 3.364 g

158. If 80% of a solution is used up, what is the decimal equivalent left?
    A. 20.0
    B. 0.2
    C. 2.0
    D. 0.02

159. Supply the missing term in the equation 3mM: 45mM :: 1 ml:X.
    A. 15 ml
    B. 0.07 ml
    C. 1 ml
    D. 1.5 ml

160. A solution has a concentration of 0.15 written on the label. What percent is this?
    A. 1.5%
    B. 150%
    C. 15%
    D. 1500%

161. Convert 1/1000 to a decimal.
    A. 0.1
    B. 0.01
    C. 0.001
    D. 0.0001

162. Using the lowest fractional reduction, how many parts of ingredient A are there to ingredient B in a 0.5 preparation?
    A. 5/10
    B. 5/100
    C. 1/2
    D. 1/20

163. How many units are needed in the proportion 10,000 u : 1 ml :: X u : 0.5 ml?
    A. 2500 units
    B. 5000 units
    C. 500 units
    D. 50,000 units

164. If a dose for a drug is 12 mg but the drug comes only as a 3 mg tablet, how many tablets are needed for the dose?
    A. 4
    B. 5
    C. 3
    D. 12

165. A prescription calls for *seventy-five hundredths* concentration of a product. How would this better be expressed as a percent?
    A. 75%
    B. 7.5%
    C. 0.075%
    D. 0.75%

166. The order calls for 20 ml of a drug. The drug comes as a 164 mg/ml concentration. What amount of drug is needed to prepare 20 ml?
    A. 3280 mg
    B. 8.2 mg
    C. 3.28 g
    D. answers A and C

167. A 5% solution contains what fraction equivalent?
    A. 1 part per 25 parts
    B. 5 parts per 10 parts
    C. 5 parts per 100 parts
    D. 50 parts per 1000 parts

168. Divide 0.1111 by 0.3333.
    A. 3.333
    B. 0.3333
    C. 30.33
    D. 3.30

169. You need 25 mg of a drug. The drug comes as 5 mg/ml; how many ml are needed to fill the order?
    A. 1 ml
    B. 25 ml
    C. 5 ml
    D. 0.5 ml

170. Multiply 0.004 by 110.012.
    A. 0.440
    B. 4.40
    C. 4.048
    D. 440.05

171. You need 4 mEq of a drug. The drug comes in 60 mEq/15 ml. How many ml are needed?
    A. 0.25 ml
    B. 1 ml
    C. 0.5 ml
    D. 1.25 ml

172. For a 20% preparation, what is a valid fractional expression?
    A. 20/100
    B. 2/10
    C. 1/5
    D. all of the above

173. Convert 112% to a decimal.
    A. 1.12
    B. 11.2
    C. 112
    D. none of the above

174. Of the following, which is the most concentrated?
    A. 50%
    B. 1.5%
    C. 70%
    D. 7%

175. In percent notation, what kind of solution is represented by 0.5?
    A. 50%
    B. 5%
    C. 0.5%
    D. 0.05%

176. Convert 0.05% to a decimal.
    A. 0.5
    B. 0.05
    C. 5.0
    D. 0.0005

177. Of the following, which is the most diluted?
    A. 50%
    B. 12.5%
    C. 1%
    D. 0.25%

178. A 10% solution has 1 part per how many parts of product?
    A. 20
    B. 1000
    C. 100
    D. 10

179. How many grams are needed to complete an order for a 1/5 preparation?
    A. 0.02 g
    B. 0.002 g
    C. 0.2 g
    D. 0.5 g

180. A 10% formulation provides how many grams of ingredient per 100 ml of a product?
   A. 0.1 g
   B. 0.01 g
   C. 10 g
   D. 1 g

181. A prescription containing a total volume of 100 ml has 5 cc given for the first dose. What percent of the total volume is this amount?
   A. 20%
   B. 10%
   C. 5%
   D. 1%

182. How many 5 ml doses are in 100 ml of product?
   A. 5
   B. 10
   C. 15
   D. 20

183. If a patient takes 75% of a 120 ml prescription, what volume is remaining?
   A. 25 ml
   B. 75 ml
   C. 30 ml
   D. 90 ml

184. If six teaspoonful doses have been given from a 4 fl. oz. prescription, what percent is this of the total prescription?
   A. 10%
   B. 25%
   C. 50%
   D. 75%

185. How is a percent volume-in-volume best defined?
   A. grams of solute in 100 milliliters of solution

   B. milliliters of solute in 100 milliliters of solution
   C. 100 milliliters of solute in any fixed quantity of solution
   D. grams of solute in 100 grams of product

186. How many ml are required to complete a prescription for 7 days for MYLANTA 30 cc pc and hs?
   A. 84 ml
   B. 630 ml
   C. 840 ml
   D. 84.0 ml

187. How is a percent weight-in-weight best defined?
   A. grams of solute in 100 grams of solution
   B. grams of solute in 100 milliliters of solution
   C. volume of solute in 100 grams of solution
   D. grams of solute in a solution that equals any precalculated percentage

188. A dose of AMOXIL is 5 ml three times a day for 10 days. How many ml is needed for the full course of treatment?
   A. 50 ml
   B. 100 ml
   C. 120 ml
   D. 150 ml

189. You have magnesium oxide 400 mg tablets on hand. On September 1, you receive a prescription that calls for 800 mg qd for the first 3 days, 400 mg BID for the next 2 days, and 400 mg qd thereafter for the remainder of September. How many tablets do you need? Remember, September has 30 days.
   A. 39
   B. 32
   C. 35
   D. 36

190. What is a ratio?
    A. the standard allowable percentage of error
    B. the relationship between two like quantities expressed as a common fraction
    C. a statistical tool
    D. a business management term referring to pricing practices

191. How many inches are in a meter?
    A. 39.37
    B. 2.54
    C. 36
    D. 15.432

192. Methylprednisolone IV has been increased to 80 mg from 60 mg. What new volume do you need from each vial containing 125 mg/5 cc?
    A. 2.4 cc
    B. 3.2 cc
    C. 0.8 cc
    D. 5.0 cc

193. How many centimeters are in an inch?
    A. 39.37
    B. 16.23
    C. 2.54
    D. 29.573

194. Which of the following measurements is the largest?
    A. g
    B. mg
    C. mcg
    D. nanogram

195. Sodium polystyrene sulfonate product is available as 15 Gm/30 ml. The product contains 20% sorbitol. How much sorbitol will the patient ingest with each 30 ml dose?

    A. 60 mg
    B. 6.0 ml
    C. 0.6 gm
    D. 6.0 gm

196. Which of the following is a measurement for liquids?
    A. mm
    B. ml
    C. gr
    D. lb

197. How many ml are needed for a 2 g dose of ANCEF if using a 500 mg/ml vial?
    A. 2
    B. 4
    C. 6
    D. 1

198. How many mg are in 3 gr?
    A. 3000
    B. 22
    C. 195
    D. 3

199. One ml is to one cc as _____ ml is to one fluid ounce.
    A. 10
    B. 1
    C. 15
    D. 30

200. An order calls for the administration of 1000 mcg of cyanocobalamine. How many milligrams will you dispense?
    A. 1 mg
    B. 10 mg
    C. 100 mg
    D. 0.1 mg

201. A Tylenol order is usually written as 10 gr q4–6h prn. What is the maxiumum dose every 24 hours in milligrams?
   A. 3900 mg
   B. 60 mg
   C. 2600 mg
   D. 650 mg

202. What do the minim, fluid drachm, and fluid ounce measure?
   A. gases
   B. fluid volume
   C. weight
   D. finished products

203. If a patient is getting 20 mEq of KCL in an hour, how long would it take for 10 mEq of KCL to be infused?
   A. 10 minutes
   B. 15 minutes
   C. 30 minutes
   D. 60 minutes

204. What is a percentage?
   A. a computation based on 10
   B. a calculation using the log scale
   C. 100
   D. an expression that indicates the quantity per hundred

205. How many milliliters of desmopressin injection are needed to fill an order requiring a patient to receive 0.2 mcg desmopressin per kg body weight when the patient weighs 150 pounds and the drug is available as 0.4 mcg per ml?
   A. 3.4 ml
   B. 120 ml
   C. 9.0 ml
   D. 34 ml

206. In household measure, how much medication should a patient take if the prescription reads, "Guaifenesin 15 cc. q4h po prn"?
   A. Take 1 teaspoonful orally every 4 hours as needed.
   B. Take 1 1/2 teaspoonsful orally every 4 hours as needed.
   C. Take 1 tablespoonful by mouth every 4 hours as needed.
   D. Take 1 ounce by mouth every 4 hours as needed.

207. How many milligrams of desmopressin acetate injection are contained in one 10 ml multiple-dose vial containing 4 mcg/ml?
   A. 40 mg
   B. 0.4 mg
   C. 4 mg
   D. 0.04 mg

208. If a 1 ml ampule of phytonadione injection contains 10 mg and the order calls for 7 mg of phytonadione, how many ml are needed to fill the order?
   A. 1.4 ml
   B. 0.7 ml
   C. 0.5 ml
   D. 0.35 ml

209. How much guaifenesin would you dispense for a 5-day supply if the prescription calls for "Guaifenesin 15 cc. q4h po prn"?
   A. 120 ml
   B. 180 ml
   C. 450 ml
   D. 480 ml

210. What does the following order mean: "2 po qam and qhs."
   A. Insert 2 suppositories rectally in the morning and at night
   B. Take 2 tablets by mouth twice a day

C. Take 1–2 tablets by mouth anytime during the day.

D. Take 2 tablets or capsules by mouth in the morning and at bedtime.

211. How many tablets are in a container holding 32500 mg of active ingredient if each tablet contains 325 mg?
A. 100
B. 50
C. 25
D. none of the above

212. How much hydrocortisone and menthol would you use in a compound for 240 ml of an emollient lotion containing 2% hydrocortisone and 1/4% menthol?
A. HC @ 480 mg menthol @ 600 mg
B. HC @ 4.8 g menthol @ 600 mg
C. HC @ 480 mg menthol @ 0.6 g
D. HC @ 48 mg menthol @ 60 mg

213. What is the cost for 24 mg of an active ingredient used in a compound if the bulk bottle of the active ingredient costs $250 per gram?
A. $9.00
B. $6.00
C. $3.00
D. $1.50

214. The average monthly use of TENORMIN is 64 tablets. It comes in 100-tablet boxes. How many boxes of 100 do you need to order for a 3-month period?
A. 3
B. 4
C. 5
D. 2

215. How many teaspoonsful are in a tablespoonful?
A. 2

B. 3
C. 4
D. 5

216. How many capsules are needed for the following script: "Amoxicillin 250 mg 1 tid for 10 days"?
A. 10
B. 20
C. 30
D. 40

217. Calculate the quantity of drug to dispense in a prescription that reads "Guaifenesin, Sig: ii tsp. q4h around the clock for 3 days."
A. 120 cc
B. 180 ml
C. 240 ml
D. 36 ml

218. A 1200 ml IV bag was hung at 0900 and is to run at 100 ml/hr. What time would the next bag be needed?
A. 1900
B. 2100
C. 2000
D. 2200

219. 4 is to *IV* as 10 is to _____.
A. L
B. M
C. X
D. C

220. Nitroglycerin is available in a variety of strengths including 1/150 gr. What is this in milligrams?
A. 6.6 mg
B. 15.0 mg
C. 0.15 mg
D. 0.4 mg

221. How many liters are in a dozen pints of dis-
    infectant?
    A. 5760 L
    B. 5.76 L
    C. 57.6 ml
    D. 576 ml

222. If a TPN order states 2 units of insulin per
    100 ml is needed, what is the total units of
    insulin needed for a 2000 ml bag?
    A. 20
    B. 30
    C. 40
    D. 50

223. A patient is taking 1 tablet of prednisone
    20 mg bid. How many doses would need to
    be filled for a 2-day supply?
    A. 1
    B. 2
    C. 3
    D. 4

224. If the dispensing fee is $5 and the price of
    100 tablets of NORVASC is $110, how
    much would a prescription for 30 tablets of
    NORVASC be?
    A. $50
    B. $48
    C. $38
    D. $33

225. You need 30 mg of gentamicin. The vial
    comes as 80 mg/ml. What is the amount in
    ml that you need?
    A. 1
    B. 0.5
    C. 0.375
    D. 0.45

226. How many cc are in 1 ml?
    A. 1
    B. 5

C. 30
D. 120

227. A 1 L IV bag is hung at 0600 and needs to
    be changed at 1400. How fast was it run-
    ning?
    A. 100 ml/hr
    B. 125 ml/hr
    C. 110 ml/hr
    D. 120 ml/hr

228. What does the Roman numeral "C"
    represent?
    A. 10
    B. 20
    C. 50
    D. 100

229. How many grams are in a kilogram?
    A. 10
    B. 100
    C. 1/1000
    D. 1000

230. What does the Roman numeral "L"
    represent?
    A. 5
    B. 20
    C. 50
    D. 100

231. How many cubic centimeters are in one
    milliliter?
    A. 1
    B. 10
    C. 100
    D. 1000

232. A dose for a drug is 5 mg/kg. A patient
    weighs 110 lbs. The drug comes in a
    100 mg/ml vial. How many ml are needed
    for this dose?
    A. 250 ml

B. 2.5 ml

C. 5 ml

D. 25 ml

233. A patient is getting a drug 500 mg bid. If the strength is increased by 20%, how much is the patient getting in one day with the increase in dosage?

A. 1000 mg

B. 2000 mg

C. 1100 mg

D. 1200 mg

234. How do you read "Nystatin s/s 5 cc q6h"?

A. Nystatin stable/suspension, 1 teaspoonful every 6 hours

B. Nystatin, swish and swallow 1 teaspoonful every 6 hours

C. Nystatin solubilized solution, 1 teaspoonful every 6 hours

D. Nystatin, saliva susceptibility, 1 teaspoonful every 6 hours

235. What information is needed in the following: "ZOFRAN 4mg q6hprn"?

A. strength

B. route of administration

C. generic name

D. reason for the drug

236. Which of the following answers is an equivalent of 1/2 ounce?

A. one tablespoonful

B. 15 cc

C. 15 ml

D. all of the above

237. A bag contains 20 mg/ml of a drug. If the bag is running at 50 ml/hr, what is the rate the bag is going in mg/hr?

A. 10

B. 100

C. 1000

D. none of the above

238. The difference between a dose of 1 "t." and 1 "T." on a prescription is the difference between _____ and _____, respectively.

A. 15 ml and 30 ml

B. titration and time (of the absorption of 1 dose)

C. 5 cc and 30 cc

D. 5 ml and 15 ml

239. What does the prefix "milli" mean?

A. 1/10

B. 1/100

C. 1/1000

D. 1000 times

240. How many ml of 50% $MgSO_4$ are needed for 500 ml of 30%?

A. 300

B. 500

C. 250

D. 400

241. What is wrong with the prescription, "Give diphenhydramine po"?

A. no strength

B. no form

C. no dosing instructions

D. all of the above

242. What is the difference between 1 oz, 30 ml, 30 cc, and 2T?

A. 2T is twice the amount of 1 oz

B. There is no difference.

C. 30 ml and 30 cc are equivalent, and 2T is double the amount of 1 oz

D. It is an irrelevant answer because there is no logical relationship among the measures.

☑answers & rationales

1.

D. Dividing 20 into 1 will give you 0.05. Multiplying it by 100% will give 5%.

2.

B. 15% is converted to a decimal by dividing by 100, giving 0.15.

3.

C. Cross-multiplying gives 50ml(X) = 200mEq(1ml). Dividing by 50ml on both sides leaves X = 4mEq.

4.

B. 12.5% is equivalent to 0.125. The number goes out to the thousandths; therefore, the fractional form is 125/1000.

5.

C. By lining up the decimal points and adding, the answer turns out to be 111.1mg.

6.

C. The fraction 1/2 is equivalent to half or 50%.

7.

B. 500 × 5.0123 yields 2506.15.

8.

D. Dividing the numerator and denominator by 25 gives 1/4.

9.

B. 12% is 12.0%. Moving the decimal point to the left two places gives 0.12.

10.

C. 15% as a decimal is 0.15 and this is the same as 15/100 and dividing both the top and bottom by 5 yields 3/20.

11.

A. Rearranging the equation, you would get (4%)(2.4mEq) = (x)(7.2mEq). Solving for x, you would get 12%.

12.

B. 3/4 is equivalent to 75% or 0.75

13.

A. 12.5% is the same as 0.125. Therefore, the fraction is 125/1000 = 1/8.

14.

C. 12.5% is 0.125

15.

C. 1.7% is 0.017

16.

D. Three quarters is equivalent to 3/4.

17.

A. 50% is one-half or 1/2

18.

C. 1/20 is equivalent to 0.05

19.

B. Rearranging the equation, (400mcg)(1ml) = (40mcg)(x). Solving for x, you get 10ml.

20.

A. 2/5 is equivalent to 0.4

21.

D. Rearranging the equation, (2.4mEq)(1ml) = (5ml)(x). Solving for x yields 0.48mEq.

22.

D. 12.5% = 0.125. This is 125/1000, dividing the numerator and denominator by 125 gives 1/8.

23.

D. 2/3 × 4/5 = 8/15. Just multiply straight across the top and bottom.

24.

C. Three-quarters is 3/4 or 75%.

25.

A. 100% − 90% = 10% or 0.1

26.

A. 25/100 is the same as saying twenty-five hundredths.

27.

A. The decimal points must be moved two places to the left first, then it would be 50/25 or 2.

28.

B. 3/5 is equivalent to dividing 5 into 3 or 0.6

29.

D. 1/2 is equivalent to 0.5. Adding in the 1 gives you 1.5.

30.

B. 1/4 is the same as having 4 divided into 1 or 0.25. Then, moving two decimal places gives you 25%.

31.

C. Rearranging the equation gives you (5000 units)(X ml) = (1250 units)(1 ml). Solving for X would yield 0.25 ml.

32.

A. Dividing 4/5 by 1/2 has to be done by first flipping the second fraction to 2/1 and then multiplying the fractions straight across, 4/5 × 2/1 = 8/5.

33.

B. 4/100 is equivalent to 100 divided into 4.00 or 0.04

34.

B. First, the fraction is the same as having 20 divided into 3.0 yielding 0.15, which is 15%.

35.

A. Rearranging the equation gives 3(27) = 9(X), solving for X gives 9.

36.

A. 5/8 is equivalent to having 8 divided into 5.0, which gives 0.625.

37.

D. Adding all three numbers gives 1.7116 g. However, none of the numbers with the unit g is correct. Therefore, moving the decimal three places to the right gives 1,711 mg.

38.

B. 20% is the same as 0.2. The expression has to be solved by multiplying 0.2 with 250, giving 50.

39.

D. Rearranging the equation yields (X mcg)(10 ml) = (1 ml)(400 mcg), solving for X gives 40 mcg.

40.

A. 7/20 is the same as having 20 divided into 7.0 or 0.35.

41.

C. Moving the decimal points over four spaces to the right gives 6875/8125 or 0.8462.

42.

D. One-tenth is the same as 1/10.

43.

C. 87% − 12% is 75%. Converting this to a decimal by moving two spaces to the left yields 0.75.

44.

C. The word expression is the same as 125/1000. Convert the fraction to a decimal by moving the decimal point, 125.0, to the left three spaces to give 0.125.

45.

B. Rearranging the problem gives (40mEq)(30ml) = (120mEq)(X). Solving for X gives 10ml.

46.

C. Two-tenths is equivalent to 2/10. As a decimal, it's 0.2. Moving the decimal point to the right two places yields 20%.

47.

D. Moving the decimal point two spaces to the right gives 150%.

48.

D. Fifteen-hundreths is 15/100. Reducing the top and bottom by a factor 5 gives 3/20.

49.

A. Moving the decimal point two spaces to the right gives 45.3%

50.

C. First, 8/40 should be reduced. Dividing by 8 on top and bottom to give 1/5 does this. 1/5 is equivalent to 0.2.

51.

D. 118ml − 23.75ml = 94.25ml

52.

A. First, 4/12 should be reduced by 4 on top and bottom. This yields 1/3, which is the same as 33%.

53.

C. Moving the decimal point two spaces to the right turns 1.05 to 105%.

54.

A. Reducing 75/100 by dividing by 25 on top and bottom yields 3/4, which is 75%.

55.

C. Rearranging the equation gives (234mg)(X) = (23.4%)(117mg). Solving for X gives 11.7%. However, the answer can be solved intuitively by realizing that X represents a percentage. Looking at the answers given, only one answer is given as a percentage; therefore, that answer must be the correct one. This should be done when possible to conserve time.

56.

B. Dividing the top and bottom by 5 gives an equation of 1/20.

57.

A. 1075 − 1.25 = −0.175. It is a negative because we are taking away a larger number from a smaller one.

58.

C. One-tenth is 1/10. The decimal equivalent is 0.1.

59.

C. Since all the answers are in grams, the first step is to convert all the units to grams. This would yield 0.45g + 5g + 3.5g = 8.95g.

60.

D. First, multiply the 350ml by 25%. This is done by changing 25% to 0.25 and then multiplying by

350ml to give 87.5ml. To convert to liters, 87.5ml should be divided by 1000 to move the decimal point three spaces to the left to give 0.087L.

61.

D. Dividing 0.3333 into 0.6667 gives 2.003.

62.

A. 2/10 can be reduced by 2 to give 1/5.

63.

A. Rearranging the problem gives (5mg)(X) = (2ml)(2mg). Solving for X gives 0.8ml.

64.

B. Reducing by 5 gives 3/20, which is the same as 0.15.

65.

D. 24.8 fl oz − 12 fl oz = 12.8 fl oz

66.

A. There are two ways to solve this problem. First, just multiplying 1/2 with 5/10 straight across gives 5/20, which is 1/4 or 25%. The second way is to realize that 5/10 is 1/2 or 50%, so the question is asking "what is half of 50%?" and the answer is 25%.

67.

D. 1 is simply 100%.

68.

C. One way to solve this is to simply convert all the anwers to percent. The good part is that all the fractions are commonly seen ones and can easily be converted to a percentage. 2/5 is 40%, which is larger than 30%. The others are 25%, 10%, and 5%, respectively, for a, b, and d.

69.

C. Rearranging the equation gives (50mEq)(4ml) = (2.5ml)(X). Solving for X gives 80mEq.

70.

D. For this, converting all the answers to a decimal then percent would be the best way. However, taking a quick glance at the answers does reveal the obvious answer of 0.07 or 7% as being the one lower than 50%.

71.

A. 1/4 is having 4 divided into 1, which is the same as 25%.

72.

C. 0.05 is in the hundredths place after the decimal point. Therefore, it is read five-hundredths.

73.

C. For this, you would have to convert all the units to grams or milligrams to decide which answers to eliminate. Converting to mg, you get 187.4 mg + 13000 mg + 276 mg = 13463.4 mg. Converting that to grams, you get 13.4634 g, giving you choice C.

74.

D. 65% is the same as 0.65 or 65/100. Reducing by 5 gives you 13/20.

75.

C. 1.25% is the same as 1 1/4; to convert to an improper fraction, the 4 is multiplied with the one then added to the 1 on the numerator and keeping the denominator the same gives 5/4.

76.

B. Converting the numbers to a percent, you would get 55%, 66%, and 62.5% for a, b, and d, respectively. Since B is 80%, that is the largest value out of the four.

77.

D. You could do one of two things: First, you could rearrange the equation and isolate X to one side. The second option is to reduce 8/16 to lowest terms by reducing by 8 to give 1/2. Either way, the answer comes out to be 2.

78.

C. The term numerically is 125/1000. Reducing by 125 gives 1/8.

79.

A. This is a straightforward problem, just remember to line up the decimal points before performing the addition function.

80.

B. Dividing 8 into 3 gives 0.375.

81.

B. Converting all the numbers to percent, you get 75%, 10%, and 35% for a, b, and d, respectively. Since C is 45%, the smallest is 10%.

82.

A. 15/100 is the same as 0.15. Converting that to a decimal, you get 15%.

83.

D. Adding all the numbers as ml you would get 127ml + 12.7ml + 1.25ml + 1000ml = 1140.95ml. Now converting to liters, you would have 1.14095L, which is both A and C.

84.

D. Reducing the numbers by 2, you would get 3/4.

85.

A. Dividing 0.5 into 0.8333, you would get 1.67.

86.

A. 45.5% is equivalent to 0.455. This would be expressed as a fraction as 455/1000.

87.

A. 1000mg − 543.1mg = 546.9mg

88.

C. First, you would need to figure out what is 15% of 200. Taking 0.15 and multiplying with the 200, you would get 30. Since the question is asking for which is the largest, the answer would be 45.

89.

D. Dividing 0.45 into 0.65, you would get 1.44, keeping the decimal point in the same place for both numbers.

90.

C. For this, you would have to perform a process of elimination. Converting all to a percent, you would get 50%, 75%, 90%, and 67% for a, b, c, and d, respectively. Since the answer must be larger than 45% and smaller than 85%, the only one that cannot fulfill this need is 90%.

91.

C. For this, it is important to remember to have three spaces to the right of the decimal point in the answer. Performing the multiplication function gives an answer of 240.960.

92.

B. Converting the answers to a percent, you would have 90%, 40%, 110%, and 80% for a, b, c, and d, respectively. Therefore, 40% would be chosen for being less than 60%.

93.

B. Dividing 10.2 into 23.75 would yield 2.33, remembering to keep the decimal point in the correct place when performing the function.

94.

C. 0.5 multipied with 3.5 would give 1.75. Converting it to a percent by moving the decimal point two spaces to the right would give 175%.

95.

A. Converting the percent to decimal numbers, you would have 13.55×4.5. Performing the operation, you would get 60.975.

96.

B. Reducing the fraction by 5 would give the lowest term of 3/20.

97.

B. Dividing 0.65 into 0.45 you would get 0.69.

98.

B. Six and five-eighths refers to having a mixed fraction of a whole number and a fraction, 6 5/8.

99.

B. Rearranging the equation, you would get $(3mMol)(X) = (150mMol)(50ml)$. Solving for X, you would get 2500ml.

100.

C. Twenty-five hundredths is 25/100, which is the same as 0.25. Converting it to a percent, you would get 25%.

101.

A. Performing the addition function, you would have to line up the decimal point so the answer would be 83.09502.

102.

A. For this, you would set up an equation of $(0.3)X = 105$. Dividing by 0.3 in order to isolate X, you would get 350.

103.

C. For this, you could multiply normally, or by multiplying any number by 0.001 would lead to moving the decimal point three spaces to the left to give 0.002.

104.

A. Five-hundredths is the same as having 5/100.

105.

C. Once again, adding up the numbers you have to keep the decimal point all lined up in order to get the correct answer of 0.491.

106.

C. 0.05 is equivalent to 5% by moving the decimal point two spaces to the right.

107.

A. Multiplying the two terms, and remembering to have three spaces after the decimal point, you would get an answer of 63.706; rounding off would give 63.71.

108.

D. Multiplying the two terms would give you 1.125. Converting to a percent, move the decimal point two spaces to the right to give 112.5%.

109.

A. Multiply the numbers and remember that you need four numbers after the decimal point to get 27.4125. Rounding off, you would get 27.41.

110.

B. Converting 25% to a decimal form would require moving the decimal point to the left two spaces, 25.0% to 0.25.

111.

B. Remembering to have two spaces after the decimal point, the answer would be 0.99.

112.

B. For this, you must remember to do the function within the parentheses first, which is multiplication, and that a negative times a positive is a negative would give you −5.25. Then, you would do the addition function to give you −0.25.

113.

A. Dividing 0.375 into 5.75 and keeping in mind the placement of the decimal point would give you 15.333.

114.

C. Since the number 0.15 is out to the hundredths place, the correct term for the number would be fifteen-hundredths.

115.

A. For this, you could rearrange the equation in order to isolate the X, but you could also realize that 25g is half of 50g and that would lead you to 50%, which is half of 100%.

116.

A. Once again, you must do the function within the parentheses first, in this case adding −15 with 20 to 5. Then, you would multiply the 5 with −45 to give you −225.

117.

D. Multiplying the equation and keeping in mind that there must be four spaces after the decimal point, you would get 2.1507, or 2.15 if you rounded it off.

118.

B. This problem requires a conversion to percentage form for all numbers. 4/5 is also 80%, so it's asking a number 56%< X< 80%. For choices a, b, c, and d, respectively, you have 40%, 65%, 55%, and 20%. The only number to fulfill both criterias is 65%.

119.

D. To convert from percent to decimal, you have to move the decimal point to the left two spaces to get 0.115.

120.

D. For 1/10, it is equivalent to the percent 10%, done by finding the decimal form and then moving the decimal to the right two spaces.

121.

C. Subtract the numbers and keep the numbers in line with each other. The correct answer is 0.015.

122.

C. This problem forces you to do a comparison. Converting everything to a percent, you would have W = 75%, 70% > X > 50%, Y < 45% and Z = 70%. Looking at these, you should figure out that W is the largest because the most any of the others can be worth is 70%.

123.

B. Converting the 3/8 to a decimal, you would have 0.375 + 0.943 + 11.21 + 27 = 39.528.

124.

C. The term one-quarter is equivalent to 25%.

125.

B. One-half is the same as 50%, so 50% + 50% is 100% or 1.

126.

C. Five-tenths is 5/10 or 0.5.

127.

B. Adding all the terms together, you would get 32.79573.

128.

D. The fractional notation for 0.15 is 15/100. Reducing it by 5, you get 3/20.

129.

B. 1/8 is equivalent to 0.125. Converting it to a percent, it would be 12.5%.

130.

D. Two-tenths is the same as 2/10.

131.

D. You could convert all terms to one unit or another. If you did it all in mg, you would have 152.5mg + 42.5mg + 1000mg + 100mg = 1295mg. Converting to grams, you would have 1.295g and converting to kg would give you 0.001295kg.

132.

B. 50% of 50% is the same as asking what is half of half, (1/2)(1/2). The answer would be 1/4, 0.25, or 25%.

133.

C. Rearranging the equation, you would have (40mEq)(X) = (2mEq)(20ml). Isolating the X, you would get 1ml.

134.

A. For 125/1000, you would need three numbers after the decimal point—0.125.

135.

A. Dividing the 3 into 2, you would get 0.666 repeating or, rounding off, you would have 0.67.

136.

D. 0.05 is in the hundredths place, so it would be 5/100.

137.

D. Adding up all the numbers, you would have 164ml, which is also the same as 0.164L.

138.

A. 0.1 is the same as 1/10, which is the lowest possible term.

139.

C. Dividing these numbers, students must stay aware of the decimal point. Since one number is longer than the other, the number on the inside when dividing should have an extra zero on the end for matching up with the longer number.

140.

D. First, you would need to find a common denominator; in this case it would be 12. The fractions you would end up adding are 3/12 + 5/12 = 8/12, which can be reduced to 2/3 or 67% (rounded up from 0.66666).

141.

B. This is simply 240 − 5.5 = 234.5 cc.

142.

A. 0.2 is the same as saying two-tenths, since the 2 is only one spot after the decimal point.

143.

D. 80% is 0.8. This would be 8/10 or reduced to 4/5.

144.

B. From the answers, you could narrow it down to choices B or D. Remembering that there are 2.2lb in 1kg, you would be able to figure out that 2kg is 4.4lb, which would make 2kg the choice. Of course, you could also convert all the choices to kg and compare the answers that way.

145.

B. 0.125 can be converted to a percent by moving the decimal point to the right two places to give 12.5%.

146.

A. Since grain is symbolized as gr, this eliminates choice D. Fifteen-hundredths can be converted to a fraction by writing it as 15/100 gr.

147.

B. 3.1g − 0.75g = 2.35g. Remember to keep the decimal points lined up in order to do this.

148.

B. 0.25 is equivalent to 25/100. Reducing by 25 gives you 1/4.

149.

C. 0.0075 is converted to a percent by moving the decimal point to the right two spaces to give you the answer of 0.75%.

150.

A. Once again, moving the decimal point to the right gives you 75%.

151.

C. 1010.101gr − 101.01 = 909.091gr. Remember to line up the decimal points.

152.

B. Five-hundredths is the same as 5/100. Since the answers are in decimal form, the correct conversion would be 0.05.

153.

C. Rearranging the equation, you get (X)(0.5g) = (4.06mEq)(25g). Solving for X, you would get an answer of 203mEq.

154.

B. 0.1 is converted to a percent by writing it as 10%.

155.

D. 35.035 − 0.35 = 34.685, remembering to line up the decimal points.

156.

D. For this, you have to convert the units to g or mg. Converting to g, you would have 35.035g −

0.00035g = 35.03465g. Converting that answer to mg, you would have 35034.65 mg.

157.

B. 11.123mg × 3mg = 33.369mg. Remember to have three numbers after the decimal point.

158.

B. If you used up 80% of a solution, that means 100% − 80%, you have only 20% left over.

159.

A. Rearranging it, you would have (3mM)(X) = (1ml)(45mM). Solving for X, you would get 15ml as the answer.

160.

C. A concentration of 0.15 is equivalent to having a percent of 15%.

161.

C. 1/1000 is the same as having a number with three spaces after the decimal point. In this case, it would be 0.001.

162.

C. Since there are only two ingredients and the preparation is 0.5, the fractional amount of one ingredient to the other is 50% or 1/2.

163.

B. Rearranging the equation, you would have (10,000u)(0.5ml) = (Xu)(1ml). Solving for X, you would have 5000u.

164.

A. A dose of 12mg would require four tablets of a 3mg tablet in order to be complete.

165.

A. Seventy-five hundredths is 0.75 or 75%.

166.

D. The ampule contains 164mg/ml and you need 20ml of it. You could simply multiply the 20ml with the 164mg/ml to eliminate the ml and give you 3280mg or 3.28g. You could also do a proportion by having Xmg/20ml = 164mg/ml and then rearranging and solving for X.

167.

C. 5% solution is the same as saying 5 parts per 100 parts since any percentage essentially means X parts of 100 parts.

168.

B. First, you should move the decimal point for both numbers to create whole numbers, 1111 divided by 3333. This would create a decimal number, 0.3333.

169.

C. Taking the 25mg, you could divide it by 5 since it's a 5mg/ml concentration to give 5ml. The other way is to set up a proportion of 25mg/x = 5mg/ml and then solve for X.

170.

A. You must remember that the answer should have six numbers after the decimal point. Once multiplied together, you have 0.440048, or 0.440 once rounded.

171.

B. 4mEq multiplied straight through with 15ml/60mEq would give you 1ml. As a proportion it would be 4mEq/X = 60mEq/15ml. Solving for X, you would have 1ml.

172.

D. 20% written as a fraction would be 20/100 or 2/10, which could go down to 1/5, so the answer would be all of the above.

173.

A. 112% is the same as writing 1.12, moving the decimal two places to the left.

174.

C. To be concentrated, the solution would have a high percent of an ingredient. In this case, the highest percentage is 70%.

175.

A. 0.5 means that the percent solution is 50%

176.

D. 0.05% can be converted to decimal form by moving the decimal two places to the left to give 0.0005.

177.

D. The meaning of a dilute solution is one where there is a low amount of solute as a part of the total solution. The lowest a number, the more dilute a solution, so the 0.25% would be the most diluted of the four listed.

178.

D. 10% can be rewritten as 1/10. So, it is 1 part per 10 parts of total solution.

179.

C. For this problem, you can take the preparation as being a total weight of 1 gram. From this view, 1/5 of 1 gram would be 0.2g.

180.

C. 10% is 10g/100ml. Since the question is asking for g in 100ml, the answer would be 10g.

181.

C. Giving 5cc is the same as 5ml. Since the total volume is 100ml, you would take 5ml/100ml to give 0.05 or 5%.

182.

D. If each dose is 5ml, you would have to divide 100ml by 5ml to give the total doses of 20.

183.

C. For this, you would need to take 75% or 0.75 and multiply it with 120ml to give 90ml. The 90ml represents the amount taken so you would take 120ml − 90ml = 30ml left.

184.

B. You would need to know that a teaspoonful is 5ml and 4 fl oz is equivalent to 120ml. Since the person took 6 tsp, that would equal 30ml. You would take 30ml/120ml to give 25%.

185.

B. The definition of percent v/v is ml of solute in 100ml of solution.

186.

C. You need to know that pc means after meals and hs is at bedtime. So, the person takes it four times a day. For 30ml per dose, the daily dose is 4 × 30ml = 120ml. Since it is needed for 7 days, you would take the 7 days and multiply by 120ml to give 840ml.

187.

A. The definition for percent w/w is grams of solute in 100g of solution.

188.

D. If the patient is to take 5ml three times a day, then that is 15ml a day. For a 10-day therapy length, you would multiply the 15ml with the 10 days to give 150ml.

189.

C. This problem is more tricky than it is difficult. You just need to take it step by step. First, 800mg qd for 3 days is the same as taking 400mg twice at one time for 3 days and that's six tablets total. For the 400mg BID or twice a day for 2 days, it is the same as four tablets. Adding that to the previous amount, you have 10 tablets total. September has 30 days. We have already been through 5 days, so 25 days

remain. If the patient is to take 400mg a day for 25 days, that would require 25 more tablets. Adding the 25 to the previous amount, you would get 35 tablets.

190.

B. As the answer states, it is a relationship between two quantities expressed as a common fraction. It is another way to express an amount.

191.

A. If you did not know the exact amount, 39.37 inches, then you could have reasoned it out. One meter is around a yard long. One yard is 3 feet, or 36 inches. Since a meter is a little more than a yard, the 39.37 would be the more logical answer based on deduction.

192.

B. You could set up a ratio in order to find the answer to this one. X/80mg = 5cc/125mg, rearranging and solving for X, you would get 3.2cc. You could also have multiplied the 80 with the concentration in a way that would isolate the cc to get you 3.2.

193.

C. For this, it is something that you just have to know, there is no real way to calculate it out. One inch is approximately 2.54 cm.

194.

A. The largest of the four is the grams or g. The others are all smaller units of weight.

195.

D. If the product is 30ml, of which 20% of it is sorbital, then (0.2)(30ml) is 6.0g of sorbital.

196.

B. The only unit of measurement for liquids listed is ml, or milliliter.

197.

B. Set up a ratio: X/2g = ml/0.5g. Solving for X, you get 4ml. Remember, 500mg = 0.5g.

198.

C. Remembering that 1gr = 65mg, you would have (3gr)(65mg/gr) = 195mg.

199.

D. You would have to know that one fluid once is equivalent to 30ml.

200.

A. 1000mcg is equivalent to 1mg because a mg is 1000 times larger than a mcg. You would have to reduce all mcg by a 1000 to get the mg equivalent, in this case 1 mg.

201.

A. For this order, the most a person can get is 10gr every 4 hours. 1gr is the same as 65mg. So, multiplying 65mg with 10gr is 650mg. Taking the 650mg and multiplying by 6 (because every 4 hours is six times a day), you would have a max of 3900mg. For Tylenol, the most an adult should get is 4000mg, or 4g, in one 24-hour period.

202.

B. All four units measure fluid volume.

203.

C. If 20mEq is going in over an hour, that means 10 mEq should go in over 30 minutes because 10 is half of 20.

204.

D. A percent is a way of measuring a quantity based on one hundred.

205.

D. First, you must convert the 150lbs to kg. This would be (150lb)(1kg/2.2lb) to give 68.2 kg. Since the dose is 0.2mcg/kg, you would multiply the 68kg with the dose to give 14mcg of the total drug. With a drug concentration of 0.4mcg/ml, you would multiply the 14mg with the 0.4mcg/ml to give you a total volume of 35ml or, if you rounded off, 34ml of drug.

206.

C. 15cc is 15ml. Since 1 tablespoonful is 15ml, the direction is "1 tablespoonful every 4 hours by mouth as needed," prn meaning "as needed."

207.

D. Take (10ml)(4mcg/ml), this would give you 40mcg or, converting to mg by dividing by 1000, 0.04mg.

208.

B. Taking (7mg)(1ml/10mg) you would get 0.7ml.

209.

C. Assuming the patient takes it every 4 hours, you would need (15ml)(6 times a day) 90ml per day. For 5 days, you would multiply 90ml with 5 days to get 450ml.

210.

D. The order means to take two tablets or capsules by mouth every morning and at bedtime.

211.

A. If a tablet contains 325mg, then a bottle of 32500mg total would contain 100 tablets (32500mg/325mg).

212.

B. If 2% of the compound is HC, you would take the (240ml)(0.02) to give 4.8g, assuming that the ingredients are in grams. For the menthol, it would be (240ml)(0.0025) to give 0.6g or 600mg.

213.

B. 24mg is 0.024g. (0.024g)($250/g) to give you $6 cost.

214.

D. If you use 64 tablets per month, you would need 192 tablets for 3 months. Since it comes as 100 tablets per box, you would need to order 2 boxes.

215.

B. One teaspoonful is 5ml, one tablespoonful is 15ml, (15ml/5ml) gives you 3 teaspoonfuls.

216.

C. 1 TID means 1 three times a day. For 10 days, this would require (10)(3) = 30 capsules.

217.

B. 2 tsp is equivalent to (2)(5ml) = 10ml. For every 4 hours, this would be (6)(10ml) = 60ml. For 3 days, this would require 180ml of drug.

218.

B. 1200ml running at 100ml/hr would last 12 hours. Since it was hung at 0900, a new bag would be needed around 2100, or 9:00 PM.

219.

C. You would need to know the Roman numerals for this. 10 is symbolized as *X*.

220.

D. 1gr is 65mg. With 1/150gr, you would have 65mg/150 = 0.4mg.

221.

B. One pint is 480ml. With a dozen pints, you would have (12)(480ml) or 5760ml. To convert to liters, you would divide by 1000 to get 5.76L.

222.

C. If you need 2 units/100ml, then you would need (2000ml)(2u/100ml) = 40 units for the bag.

223.

D. Taking a tablet twice a day would require two tablets multiplied by 2 days, which is four.

224.

C. 100 tabs/$110 = 30 tabs/X, solving for X you get $33 and adding the $5 dispensing fee would bring the final total to $38 for 30 tablets.

225.

C. 30mg/X = 80mg/ml, solving for X, you would get 0.375ml.

226.

A. 1cc is equivalent to 1ml.

227.

B. From 0600 to 1400, that is a total of 8 hours. For a 1L bag to run out by 1400, it would mean that it ran at 1000ml/8hr = 125ml/hr.

228.

D. The Roman numeral C is equivalent to 100.

229.

D. 1kg is equal to 1000 grams.

230.

C. Fifty is represented by the letter L.

231.

A. 1 cubic cm is equivalent to 1 ml.

232.

B. Converting 110lbs to kg, you would get (110lbs/2.2lbs) 50kg. Multiplying (5mg/kg)(50), you would have 250mg(ml/100mg) = 2.5ml.

233.

D. 500mg increased by 20% would give a new dose of (500mg)(0.2) = 100mg plus 500mg of the original dose would give you 600mg twice a day, for a total dose of 1200mg.

234.

B. This reads "Nystatin swish and swallow 1 teaspoonful every 6 hours."

235.

B. The order is missing the route of administration. ZOFRAN can be given by mouth or by injection.

236.

D. One ounce is 30ml. Half of that is 15ml, which is 15cc and one tablespoonful.

237.

C. For this, you would take (20mg/ml)(50ml/hr) = 1000mg/hr.

238.

D. 1t is 5ml and 1 T is 15ml.

239.

C. "Milli" means 1/1000.

240.

A. You would have to set this up as a concentration-volume problem, (500ml)(30%) = (X)(50%). Solving for X, you would get 300ml.

241.

D. The order is missing the strength (25mg or 50mg), the form (capsule or tablet), and the instructions on how to take the drug.

242.

B. There is no difference between the four. 2T is 30ml and 1 oz is also 30ml and, of course, 30 cc is also 30ml.

3 Pharmacy and Medical Terminology

chapter objectives

Students will demonstrate knowledge of:

➤ The various medical and pharmaceutical abbreviations commonly used in practice

➤ The various medical and pharmaceutical acronyms commonly used in practice

➤ The various medical and pharmaceutical jargons used in practice

➤ The various medical and pharmaceutical symbols used in practice

DIRECTIONS Each of the questions or incomplete statements below is followed by suggested answers or completions. Select the **one answer** that is best in each case.

1. A prescription for "hydrocortisone 1 percent ointment, apply TID" would most likely be written as which of the following?
   A. HC 1% oint. 3 Xid
   B. HC 1% ung. 3 id
   C. HC 1% oint. TID
   D. HC 1% oint. TOD

2. The acronym "CHF" refers to which of the following?
   A. congenital heart fibrillation
   B. conductive heart failure
   C. congestive heart failure
   D. cardiovascular hemostatic failure

3. The CII refers to which of the following?
   A. cardiovascular drugs
   B. compounded drugs
   C. a governmental payment agency
   D. controlled drug class 2

4. What does the term "neb" mean on an order?
   A. neutralization
   B. nearly equal
   C. not enabling breathing
   D. nebulizer

5. METFORMIN is an antidiabetic medication. Which of the following would be in the same general drug class as METFORMIN?
   A. ORUDIS
   B. PREVACID
   C. GLYSET
   D. TRICOR

6. How would a prescriber write the directions for "zolpidem 5 mg at bedtime if needed"?
   A. zolpidem 5 mg qhs prn
   B. zolpidem 5 mg qhs ad
   C. zolpidem 5 mg q 10 P.M.ad.lib
   D. zolpidem 5 mg qhsqs

7. What does "U.D." mean when written on a prescription?
   A. for rectal use only
   B. use as directed by physician
   C. for right ear
   D. use only during waking hours

8. What does the designation "SMZ" represent?
   A. sargramostim
   B. scopolamine
   C. sulfamethoxazole
   D. simvastatin

9. Which of the following forms of injection is usually used to administer insulin?
   A. IV
   B. SC
   C. IM
   D. IC

10. DIOVAN, ATACAND, and MICARDIS are classified in what type of antihypertensive class of drugs?
    A. calcium channel blockers
    B. ACE inhibitors
    C. angiotensin II receptor antagonists
    D. alpha-blockers

11. Seen often in compounding, ad. refers to
    _____.
    A. advance
    B. adhere
    C. before drying
    D. to, or up to

12. What does the designation "TMP" represent?
    A. triamterene
    B. trimethoprim
    C. trimeprazine
    D. triamcinolone

13. How would a prescription for "penicillin 500 milligrams immediately, and 250 milligrams four times a day" most likely be written by the prescriber?
    A. penicillin 500 mg at first, then 250 mg Q.O.D.
    B. penicillin 500 mg STAT, 250 mg QID
    C. penicillin 500 mg now, 250 mg 4xid
    D. penicillin 500 mg at once, then 250 mg QD

14. The abbreviation a.d. refers to which one?
    A. right eye
    B. left ear
    C. right ear
    D. both ears

15. What does a.c. stand for?
    A. before meals
    B. equal concentrations
    C. before withholding
    D. alternating concentrations

16. Which of the following is not a common abbreviation for a lab test?
    A. CBC
    B. CMV
    C. T & C
    D. H & H

17. How would the prescription for "sucralfate one gram four times a day before meals and at bedtime" be written?
    A. sucralfate 1 g QXd ac and hs
    B. sucralfate 1 g 4id ac and hs
    C. sucralfate 1 g QOD ac and hs
    D. sucralfate 1 g QID ac and hs

18. What is the hospital category of drugs designated as PRN?
    A. patient restriction on narcotics
    B. medications that must be refrigerated because of a short expiration date

C. refers to the method used to order the drug from the vendor
D. medications not routinely used on a specific schedule, but only when needed by the patient

19. What is the meaning of "dys" in the word dyspnea?
    A. difficult
    B. lacking
    C. slow
    D. very little

20. Hospital pharmacies may adopt for specific drugs an automatic stop-order policy usually designated by what acronym?
    A. ASOP
    B. STOP
    C. ASO
    D. AUTOSTOP

21. What are we referring to when we speak of a drug formulary for a hospital?
    A. a listing of drugs selected by the hospital P&T committee for inclusion in a pharmacy's inventory of drugs
    B. a directory of formulas that make up each drug
    C. a compounding directory
    D. a list of forms used to order various types of drugs such as controlled substances and alcohol

22. The root "vaso" in vasoconstrictor can denote drugs that affect what part of the anatomy?
    A. heart
    B. blood cells
    C. blood vessels
    D. lymph nodes

23. To what does the DEA refer?
    A. Date of Exclusion Application

B. Drug Enforcement Administration

C. Drug Entry Alert

D. Drug Evaluation Agency

24. What is ambulatory care?

A. the care provided to a patient in an ambulance

B. the care provided to only walking patients

C. health services provided on an outpatient basis

D. health services given to bedridden patients

25. What would a prescription for "naphazoline eye drops, two drops in each eye twice a day when needed for redness" look like?

A. naphazoline oph, 2 gtts OS BD prn redness

B. naphazoline oph, 2 gtts OU BID prn redness

C. naphazoline Otic, 2 gtts OU BID prn redness

D. naphazoline Otic 2 gtts od BD prn redness

26. What is the meaning of "glyco" in the word glycosuria?

A. sour

B. salty

C. sweetness

D. tartness

27. It is important to read q.i.d. and q.o.d. directions carefully because

A. q.i.d. is four times a day, q.o.d. is every other day.

B. q.i.d. is every evening, q.o.d. is every day.

C. q.i.d. is three times a day, q.o.d. is four times a day.

D. q.i.d. is four times a day, q.o.d. is day or night.

28. What is bacteremia?

A. a treatment for bacterial infection

B. bacterial infection of the blood

C. bacterial invasion of the intestine

D. diarrhea

29. How many doses can be given during a *q2hprn* schedule?

A. 12

B. 4

C. 24

D. 3

30. Rhinitis is usually a seasonal ailment. What part of the body is affected?

A. nose

B. mouth

C. eyes

D. ears

31. Another term for "hyperalimentation" solution is what?

A. fats

B. LVP

C. SVP

D. TPN

32. Drugs used to treat dermatitis are treating what condition?

A. nasal polyps

B. ringing in the ears

C. inflamed eyes

D. inflammation of the skin

33. The difference between the p.o. and p.r. routes of administration is:

A. p.o. is by mouth, p.r. is rectally

B. p.o. is rectally, p.r. is by mouth

C. p.o. is parenterally, p.r. is enterally

D. p.o. is topically, p.r. is by mouth

34. What part of the anatomy is affected by nephrotoxicity?
    A. the liver
    B. the heart
    C. the spleen
    D. the kidneys

35. The abbreviation "DNR" means what?
    A. direct nasal route
    B. do not rehab
    C. do not resuscitate
    D. diverticulitis narrowing rupture

36. The label should tell the patient to take a prescription q3h w.a.
    A. every 3 hours with antibiotics
    B. every 3 hours with water
    C. every 3 hours while awake
    D. every 3 hours as needed

37. What is the meaning of "per" in percutaneous?
    A. puncture
    B. soft
    C. pliable
    D. section of

38. By which route is a supp. given?
    A. p.o.
    B. p.r.
    C. q.d.
    D. s.a.

39. What is the meaning of "meta" in metabolism?
    A. minute
    B. false
    C. transformation
    D. deficient

40. STAT or stat on the prescription order means?
    A. statistically

B. Saturday dose
C. now, immediately, or at once
D. list the name of the drug

41. What is the meaning of "hypo" in hyponatremia?
    A. deficiency
    B. excessive
    C. dangerous
    D. drug interaction

42. Of the following, what does the acronym "IV" mean?
    A. intravenous
    B. induce ventilation
    C. infectious virus
    D. inflamed veins

43. The acronym "IM" found on the patient's orders means
    A. increase mobility
    B. intestinal mucosa
    C. inflamed muscle
    D. intramuscular

44. How would you describe the urine output using the meaning of "poly" in polyuria?
    A. deficient
    B. sweet odor
    C. excessive
    D. burning

45. A nonsedating antihistamine medication to control allergies that you would find OTC is
    A. ALLEGRA
    B. ZYRTEC
    C. CLARINEX
    D. CLARITIN

46. LOVENOX is sometimes given for prevention of DVT. What is DVT?
    A. deep vein thrombosis
    B. deep venous thrombin

C. direct vein temperature

D. direct vein throbbing

47. Which abbreviation does not belong in the following group?

A. tab.

B. syr.

C. susp.

D. subq.

48. Which of the following is not a medical diagnostic test?

A. CAT scan

B. ultrasound

C. cardiac tamponade

D. stress test

49. "Angi" in angioplasty tells us that this procedure relates to what part of the anatomy?

A. heart

B. liver

C. blood vessels

D. kidneys

50. Which of the following does not belong?

A. PZI

B. PCN

C. TCN

D. gent

51. The "gingi" in gingivitis refers to an inflammation of what part of the anatomy?

A. gums

B. teeth

C. throat

D. tongue

52. The term "pre-eclampsia" means?

A. hypertension due to unknown causes

B. constriction of uterus walls during labor

C. infection of unknown origin

D. hypertension occurring from pregnancy

53. Which of the following best describes the root part "cyte" in the word hematocyte?

A. cell

B. color

C. thickness

D. flowability

54. What does the acronym "g/d" mean?

A. grams per dose

B. gastrointestinal disorder

C. grams per day

D. granuloma dissection

55. What information is provided by the NDC numbering system?

A. the manufacturer

B. the product name, strength, and dosage form

C. the packaging size

D. all of the above

56. The integumentary system includes words such as dermatitis. What does the common root "derma" mean?

A. skin

B. nails

C. hair

D. breasts

57. Which of the following is/are some designations used by manufacturers to indicate extended or long-acting dosage forms?

A. SR

B. SA

C. CD

D. all of the above

58. The "nephr" refers to what part of the genitourinary system?

A. liver

B. spleen

C. kidney

D. bladder

59. What does the acronym "GI" mean?
    A. gastric infusion
    B. gastrointestinal
    C. gallbladder inflammation
    D. gum infection

60. Which of the following answers best describes the number to be dispensed?
    A. DTD
    B. disp
    C. #
    D. all of the above

61. The common root "osteo" refers to what part of the musculoskeletal system?
    A. bone
    B. tendon
    C. skull
    D. muscle

62. Which of the following acronyms or abbreviations on the prescription alerts us to the directions?
    A. AQ. DIST
    B. DTD
    C. SIG.
    D. STAT

63. The word arthritis can easily be dissected into "arthr" and "itis." Knowing that "itis" refers to an inflammation, which part of the skeletal system is described by "arthr"?
    A. tendons
    B. cartilage
    C. joint
    D. muscle

64. The drug TIAZAC has the generic of
    A. tolteradine
    B. verapamil
    C. diltiazem
    D. terazosin

65. Both "pneumo-" and which other common root refer to lungs?
    A. broncho-
    B. laryn-
    C. pulmo-
    D. rhin-

66. What do the IM, IV, and SC routes of administration have in common about how drugs are administered?
    A. parenterally
    B. orally
    C. in larger volumes
    D. as admixtures

67. How is the label for "Instill two gtts. ou BID" typed out for the patient?
    A. Instill 2 ophthalmic disks in both eyes twice a day.
    B. Instill 2 drops in both eyes twice a day.
    C. Instill 2 drops in each ear twice a day.
    D. Instill 2 drops in the left ear twice a day.

68. If a patient is diagnosed as having schizophrenia, which of the following drugs would he/she likely be prescribed for that particular condition?
    A. SPORANOX
    B. SEROQUEL
    C. SUCRALFATE
    D. SEREVENT

69. What does the acronym "ACE" found on a patient's orders mean?
    A. angiotensin converting enzyme
    B. abdominal extension
    C. atrophic cardiac exacerbation
    D. arterial and cardiac evaluation

70. If a patient is "hypokalemic," what does the term mean?
    A. low sodium
    B. low potassium

C. low calcium

D. low bicarbonate

71. The designation "as" means

    A. left ear

    B. right nostril

    C. right eye

    D. right ear

72. What does "CSF" stand for?

    A. cardiosuprafluid

    B. common supportive footwear

    C. cerebral skeletal form

    D. cerebrospinal fluid

73. Ophthalmic is to eye as _____ is to liver.

    A. renal

    B. hepatic

    C. digestive

    D. pulmonary

74. Otic is to ear as renal is to _____.

    A. liver

    B. eye

    C. kidney

    D. heart

75. What does the abbreviation "R/O" mean?

    A. recovering order

    B. receiving order

    C. regarding operation

    D. rule out

76. The acronym "UTI" is found on the patient's orders. What does it mean?

    A. intrathecal infusion

    B. urinary tract infection

    C. upper thoracic infection

    D. undiagnosed thyroid infection

77. A condition is noted by what suffix?

    A. ectasis

B. itis

C. pathy

D. malacia

78. How is a dose taken s.l. administered?

    A. under the tongue

    B. in the cheek cavity

    C. sublingually

    D. answers A and C

79. The acronym "GERD" is found on a patient's orders. What does it mean?

    A. gastroesophageal reflux disease

    B. geriatric evaluation for refractory dementia

    C. general evaluation by registered dietician

    D. gait evaluation required daily

80. What is the meaning of "cata" in catabolism?

    A. buildup

    B. transformation

    C. breakdown

    D. minute

81. PROZAC is to fluoxetine as _____ is to filgrastim.

    A. NEURONTIN

    B. NEBCIN

    C. NEUPOGEN

    D. NORCURON

82. MAALOX is considered to be what type of liquid?

    A. suspension

    B. solution

    C. emulsion

    D. none of the above

83. What is the term given to the opening of a needle through which fluid is drawn?

    A. tip

    B. bevel

    C. shaft

    D. port

84. In the word erythrocyte, what does "erythro-" mean?
    A. deficient
    B. redness
    C. abundant
    D. pallor

85. Which of the following is NOT a common IV fluid bag that is premixed from the manufacturer?
    A. D5LR
    B. D5NS
    C. D12.5
    D. 3%NS

86. Which of the following drugs is considered to be an OTC?
    A. REGLAN
    B. PHENERGAN
    C. CELEBREX
    D. ALEVE

87. What does the acronym "MDI" represent?
    A. medical diagnosis inquiry
    B. measured-drug inhaler
    C. physician internist
    D. metered-dose inhaler

88. What is the term given for a disease characterized by irregularly shaped red blood cells?
    A. hemophilia
    B. sickle cell
    C. rigid cell
    D. stem cell

89. The acronym "DNA" is found on the patient's orders. What does it mean?
    A. deoxyribonucleic acid
    B. do not activate
    C. diphenhydramine
    D. do not aspirate

90. What does "DT" stand for?
    A. delirium tremens
    B. delirium tremors
    C. dead tissues
    D. diagnostic tests

91. What is the common cause of "DT"?
    A. alcoholic withdrawal
    B. cancerous growth
    C. common result of aging
    D. seizures

92. What does the acronym "COPD" mean?
    A. complete official position description
    B. continue observation of patient depression
    C. cancel out peripheral dilation
    D. chronic obstructive pulmonary disease

93. The abbreviation a.u stands for
    A. each eye
    B. left eye
    C. left ear
    D. each ear

94. In the word bradycardia, what does "brady" mean?
    A. accelerated
    B. slow
    C. nonreversible
    D. deficient

95. The acronym "CNS" is found on a patient's orders. What does it mean?
    A. continue normal saline
    B. clear nasal sinuses
    C. central nervous system
    D. cancel neonatal screening

96. The common root "neuro-" refers to which part of the anatomy?
    A. nerve
    B. mind

C. spinal cord

D. brain

97. What does HCO₃ represent?

    A. hemophilus b conjugate vaccine

    B. bismuth

    C. bicarbonate

    D. hetastarch

98. What does Mg represent?

    A. magnesium hydroxide

    B. magnesium

    C. magnesium sulfate

    D. manganese

99. If a patient is getting the drug PLETAL, what part of the body would this have an effect on?

    A. joints

    B. muscles

    C. blood

    D. eyes

100. What does Ca represent?

    A. calcium

    B. calcitonin

    C. calcitriol

    D. calcium carbunale

101. The suffices "-algia" and "-dynia" refer to which type of symptom?

    A. fever

    B. headache

    C. pain

    D. constipation

102. What is the name of the hood used to compound nonchemotherapeutic drugs called?

    A. vertical flow hood

    B. horizontal flow hood

    C. compounding hood

    D. aseptic preparation hood

103. The suffix "-oma" in a word often denotes which of the following?

    A. a softening

    B. a tumor

    C. a condition

    D. an inflammation

104. What does Na represent?

    A. naproxen

    B. saline

    C. sodium chloride

    D. sodium

105. What does the acronym "mg/kg/dose" mean?

    A. magnesium per kilogram dose

    B. manganese per kilogram of body weight per dose

    C. milligrams per kilogram of body weight per dose

    D. milligrams per kilogram of drug per dose

106. The suffix "-malacia" is most closely associated with which of the following?

    A. swelling

    B. malnutrition

    C. flowing

    D. softening

107. What does K represent?

    A. potassium phosphate

    B. potassium gluconate

    C. potassium

    D. ketaconazole

108. The acronym "NSAIDs" is found on a patient's orders. What does it mean?

    A. nonstable AIDS patient

    B. no susceptibility to AIDS

    C. normal saline for AIDS patients

    D. nonsteroidal anti-inflammatory drugs

109. What does Li represent?

    A. liothyronine

    B. lithium

    C. liotrix

    D. lisinopril

110. The suffix for inflammation is described by which of the following?

    A. -cele

    B. -itis

    C. -mania

    D. -rrhea

111. What does the acronym "OTC" mean?

    A. over-the-counter

    B. observed technical count

    C. ophthalmic treatment considered

    D. outside the curriculum

112. What does the term "PCA" stand for?

    A. patient-controlled analgesia

    B. patient-calibrated analysis

    C. partially collapsed atrium

    D. perinial circumvented artherosclerosis

113. The "rhin" in rhinitis describes this inflammation to be associated with what part of the respiratory system?

    A. windpipe

    B. lungs

    C. larynx

    D. nose

114. Which drug listed below would be classified as a benzodiazepine?

    A. ULTRAM

    B. SERAX

    C. BUSPAR

    D. MAXITROL

115. The prefix "litho" has the meaning of what?

    A. psychosis

    B. depression

    C. fatigue

    D. calcification

116. As "psych" refers to the mind, "cere" refers to which part of the nervous system?

    A. the head

    B. brain

    C. nerve

    D. vertebrae

117. What does the abbreviation "PCN" mean?

    A. post-care nutrition

    B. platelet count plus neutrophils

    C. penicillin

    D. piperacillin

118. What does the acronym "LMWH" stand for?

    A. lactulose magnesium water hydrolysis

    B. left meniscule weight hyperextension

    C. low molecular weight heparin

    D. lower mid-waist hernia

119. What part of the musculoskeletal system is affected by pain when referring to "chondrodynia"?

    A. joints

    B. skull

    C. tendons

    D. cartilage

120. The acronym "PUD" found on a patient's orders means

    A. provide unit dose

    B. plicamycin-uracil-dactinomycin regimen

    C. pathogenic ureter disorder

    D. peptic ulcer disease

121. What is the difference between homeostasis and hemostasis?

    A. no difference

    B. Homeostasis refers to a balance in the body's physiologic systems, and hemostasis refers to properties of vasocon-striction and blood coagulation.

C. Hemostasis refers to a balance in the body's physiologic systems, and home-ostasis refers to properties of vasocon-striction and blood coagulation.

D. Hemostasis refers to blood stability and homeostasis to blood coagulation.

122. Knowing that "dynia" refers to pain, drugs used to alleviate mastodynia affect which part of the anatomy?

A. jaw

B. breast

C. neck

D. mastoid bone

123. What does the term "NTG" mean?

A. nitroglycerin

B. nipride

C. no telemetry given

D. not tolerating gases

124. What does the acronym "RA" mean?

A. rheumatoid arthritis

B. right atrium

C. regional ascites

D. refractory anemia

125. Some drug side effects may include glossi-tis. The "gloss" refers to what part of the anatomy?

A. vocal cords

B. tongue

C. cheeks

D. salivary glands

126. What most commonly follows the "#" sym-bol on a prescription?

A. a quantity

B. a time

C. a schedule

D. a weight

127. Drugs that have a renal impact have an ef-fect on which organ of the body?

A. pancreas

B. liver

C. lungs

D. kidney

128. The initials "XL" that appears after a drug name means

A. extra large tablet

B. extended release

C. experimental drug

D. extra strength formulation

129. The acronym "SOB" found on the patient's orders means

A. standard operational billing

B. shortness of breath

C. signs of bacteremia

D. start observing breathing

130. "Emia" in hyperemia and "hem" in hemapoiesis refers to what part of the anatomy?

A. spleen

B. blood

C. veins

D. arteries

131. Which of the following is a designation you will not find on a prescription order?

A. #

B. Disp.

C. Sig:

D. NB

132. Which of the following professional li-censes is not allowed to prescribe medica-tion?

A. MD

B. PA

C. CRNA

D. DDS

133. The "gastr" in gastritis refers to what part of the anatomy?
    A. liver
    B. kidney
    C. intestines
    D. stomach

134. What does the acronym "SSRI" mean?
    A. Standard System of Regional Infusion
    B. subsequent signs of respiratory inhibition
    C. selective serotonin reuptake inhibitor
    D. saturated solution of riboflavin injection

135. DOSS or DSS is used as what type of medication?
    A. laxative agent
    B. diabetic hypoglycemic agent
    C. antiemetic drug
    D. antidiarrheal drug

136. The root "cardium" in pericardium refers to what part of the anatomy?
    A. lungs
    B. aortic artery
    C. jugular vein
    D. heart

137. Diuretics affect the kidneys as cardiac drugs affect the _____?
    A. liver
    B. heart
    C. immune system
    D. gallbladder

138. By reading the word tachycardia, what do we know from the prefix "tachy" about the beating of the heart?
    A. slowed
    B. accelerated
    C. irregular
    D. lacking

139. What does the acronym "TCAs" found on a patient's orders mean?
    A. thoracic congested areas
    B. tetracycline agents
    C. tertiary catheter administration
    D. tricyclic antidepressants

140. Of the following listed, which drug would have the strength written as "units"?
    A. enoxaparin
    B. warfarin
    C. heparin
    D. ticlopidine

141. The prefix "semi" gives what meaning to the word semipermeable?
    A. total
    B. block
    C. unmeasurable
    D. partial

142. Which of the following organizations would be more concerned with the operations of an institutional/hospital pharmacy?
    A. JCAHO
    B. DEA
    C. OSHA
    D. DPS

143. In the word pericarditis, what best describes the closest meaning for the prefix "peri?"
    A. within
    B. around
    C. through
    D. of close proximity

144. What does the abbreviation "TCN" mean?
    A. tetracycline
    B. total care nutrition
    C. tetracaine
    D. ticarcillin

145. What could we deduce from a report that notes glycosuria?
    A. There is excessive urine output.
    B. Sugar is found in the urine.
    C. Urine output has diminished.
    D. Stools show blood content.

146. What drug is commonly used during a PTCA procedure?
    A. abciximab
    B. adenosine
    C. acyclovir
    D. acarbose

147. A person suffering from dyspnea shows what problem?
    A. difficulty in breathing
    B. snoring
    C. wheezing
    D. heart attack

148. The difference between C and c in a prescription is
    A. C means carefully, c means with.
    B. C means 100, c means caution.
    C. C means compound, c means capsules.
    D. C means 100, c means with.

149. Where is the bleeding occurring when located intracranially?
    A. around the heart
    B. within the eye
    C. around the spleen
    D. within the skull

150. Before filling a precription for the drug VICODIN, what should always be verified first?
    A. DEA number of doctor
    B. address of doctor
    C. phone number of doctor's office
    D. spelling of the doctor's name

151. What is the normal unit of measurement for BSA?
    A. cm^3
    B. inches
    C. ml
    D. m^2

152. What does b.i.d. mean in the directions, "Take 1 tablet b.i.d."?
    A. before ingesting diet
    B. before bedtime
    C. twice a day
    D. none of the above

153. Before you mix and prepare any antineoplastic drug, what should you always be wearing?
    A. double gloves
    B. gown buttoned in the back
    C. latex boots
    D. A and B

154. A drug target is most closely related to
    A. the liver
    B. the cytochrome P 450 system
    C. a receptor site
    D. the circulatory system

155. How many "qhs" doses can be given "qd"?
    A. 24
    B. 4
    C. 3
    D. 1

156. Which of the following drugs would NOT require frequent blood levels?
    A. DILANTIN
    B. DEPAKOTE
    C. ERYTHROCIN
    D. THEO-DUR

157. What is MedWatch?

   A. a service to monitor polypharmacy in the elderly

   B. a service to watch community pharmacies to prevent crime

   C. a reporting program available to health care providers to report adverse events that can pose a serious health threat

   D. a device that signals the need for prescribed medication

✓answers & rationales

1.

C. Hydrocortisone is abbreviated HC and the strength would be written 1% with ointment abbreviated oint.

2.

C. CHF refers to congestive heart failure.

3.

D. CII refers to controlled drug class 2, which would include morphine, meperidine, and oxycontin.

4.

D. "Neb" refers to hand-held nebulizer, an instrument used to help patients breath and to administer the drugs albuterol and ipratropium for treatment of breathing difficulties.

5.

C. GLYSET is classified in the general class of antidiabetic agent, same as METFORMIN.

6.

A. For this order, the "at bedtime if needed" would be written "qhs prn."

7.

B. "UD" usually stands for "as directed" on a prescription.

8.

C. "SMZ" represents the drug "sulfamethoxazole."

9.

B. Insulin is given SC, or subcutaneously.

10.

C. The three drugs listed are all part of the class called angiotensin II receptor antagonists.

11.

D. ad in compounding terms refers to adding an ingredient "to or up to" a certain amount.

12.

B. "TMP" represents the drug trimethoprim. TMP-SMZ are the ingredients in BACTRIM or Co-trimazole.

13.

B. Penicillin 500mg STAT, then 250mg qid.

14.

C. a.d. refers to right ear.

15.

A. a.c. stands for "before meals."

16.

B. CMV is cytomegalovirus; T&C is type and cross and used when blood is needed for a transfusion; CBC is complete blood count and H&H is hemoglobin and hematocrit.

17.

D. The amount of "1 gram" is 1 g and "four times a day before meals and at bedtime" would be QID ac and hs.

18.

D. PRN is a designation for drugs given only when the patient needs it, not on a routine daily schedule.

19.

A. "Dys" has the meaning of difficult. In this case, the word means difficulty in breathing.

20.

C. Automatic Stop Order is abbreviated ASO.

21.

A. A drug formulary is a listing of drugs that was approved by the P&T committee to be included in the inventory of a hospital. The amount of different drugs and different types of drugs to be carried is dependent on each institution's needs and overall usage of a drug.

22.

C. "Vaso" refers to the blood vessels. In this case, the word has the meaning of constriction of the blood vessels.

23.

B. DEA stands for Drug Enforcement Administration. This branch of the U.S. government is mainly involved in the distribution, transportation, and use of controlled drugs.

24.

C. Ambulatory care is a term to designate health services provided on an outpatient basis.

25.

B. "Two drops in each eye twice a day when needed for redness" would be written as "2 gtts OU BID prn redness" and it would be written "oph" for ophthalmic. The "otic" is a designation for the ear, not the eye.

26.

C. "Glyco" stands for sweetness. In this case, the term means excretion of sugar in the urine.

27.

A. QID stands for four times a day while QOD means every other day. If the two were misread for each other, then there would be a major dispensing error.

28.

B. Bacteremia means that there has been a bacterial infection of the blood.

29.

A. "Q2hprn" means a patient can get a dose every 2 hours. Since there are 24 hours in a day, the total maximum number of doses would be 12.

30.

A. Rhinitis refers to the inflammation of the nasal passages of the nose.

31.

D. Hyperalimentation is an older term referring to TPNs, or total parental nutrition, which is given to patients who are in serious condition and are not able to eat solid food.

32.

D. Dermatitis means an inflammation of the skin.

33.

A. The p.o. route refers to oral administration while the p.r. route refers to rectal administration.

34.

D. Nephrotoxicity refers to damaging of the kidneys.

35.

C. The term "DNR" refers to "do not resuscitate." The term is sometimes found on charts of patients who have terminal illnesses and do not wish to be revived if they go into a traumatic event.

36.

C. Q3h w.a. means "every 3 hours while awake."

37.

A. "Per" refers to puncture. In this case, the term means puncture of the skin tissue.

38.

B. Supp is shorthand form for suppository and it is given rectally or p.r.

39.

C. "Meta" means transformation. In this case, the term means to transform food into energy and needed components for the functioning of the body.

40.

C. STAT on a prescription indicates that the patient needs the medication now, immediately, or at once. This is used to get the attention of the pharmacy and to make that prescription a priority in the filling process.

41.

A. "Hypo" means deficiency. Hyponatremia means a deficiency in sodium.

42.

A. "IV" stands for intravenous. It is used for drugs specifically indicated to be given by injection into a vein.

43.

D. "IM" means intramuscular, which is the process of giving medication within muscle and does not go directly into the veins.

44.

C. "Poly" means excessive. For the term polyuria, it means excessive production of urine.

45.

D. CLARITIN is the only drug of the four listed that is available OTC.

46.

A. "DVT" means deep vein thrombosis. This condition refers to having a blood clot in the blood vessels. LOVENOX is a drug given to prevent this occurrence.

47.

D. Subq means subcutaneous and it is a route of administration by injection. The other routes are all oral.

48.

C. Cardiac tamponade is a condition where the heart is compressed due to increased fluid in the pericardium. The other three are all medical tests used to help diagnose medical conditions.

49.

C. "Angi" relates to the blood vessels. In this case, angioplasty is a process whereby the blood vessels are opened up through an invasive technique.

50.

A. PZI is the only one of the four that is not an antibotic of some type. PZI is protamine zinc insulin. PCN is penicillin, TCN is tetracycline, and gent is short for gentamicin.

51.

A. "Gingi" refers to the gums. Therefore, gingivitis refers to inflammation of the gums.

52.

D. Pre-eclampsia refers to a hypertensive condition occurring from pregnancy or a recent pregnancy.

53.

A. "Cyte" refers to cell. In this case, hematocyte means blood cells.

54.

C. "g/d" means grams per day. This indicates the amount of medication a patient is to receive on a daily basis.

55.

D. Each of the three different sets of numbers corresponds to manufacturer, product name, strength, dosage form, and packaging size.

56.

A. "Derma" means skin. Dermatitis means inflammation of the skin.

57.

D. All of the three listed are common ways in which drug manufacturers designate extended or long-acting dosage forms.

58.

D. "Nephr" refers to the kidney, nephrotoxicity.

59.

B. "GI" means gastrointestinal.

60.

D. All of the four choices listed can be used to designate the quantity of drug to be dispensed. "DTD" means dispense total dose, "disp" means dispense, and the "#" refers to number.

61.

A. "Osteo" is a term that refers to the bones of the body.

62.

C. SIG is the abbreviation mostly used to designate the instructions of a prescription. The term actually has the meaning "let it be marked."

63.

C. "Arthr" refers to the joints of the body. Therefore, arthritis is inflammation of the joints.

64.

C. TIAZAC is a drug used to control blood pressure that has the generic name of diltiazem.

65.

C. "Pulmo" is also a term that refers to the lungs. "Broncho" may sound like it relates to the lungs but it refers to the windpipe. "Laryn" refers to the vocal cords while "rhin" refers to the nasal passages.

66.

A. IM, IV, and SC are all parenteral routes of administration.

67.

B. The direction on the label is read "instill 2 drops in both eyes twice a day."

68.

B. SEROQUEL is in the class of drugs known as the atypical antipsychotic agents. A patient with schizophrenia or another psychosis condition could be prescribed this drug.

69.

A. "ACE" is the acronym for a substance called "angiotensin converting enzyme," which causes hypertension in some patients.

70.

B. "Hypokalemic" means having low levels of potassium in the body.

71.

D. "as" means left ear.

72.

D. "CSF" means "cerebral spinal fluid."

73.

B. Hepatic is a term relating to the liver.

74.

C. Renal is a term relating to conditions and events of the kidney.

75.

D. "R/O" is an abbreviation for "rule out." This term appears on physician orders as "R/O MI," for example. This means that a physician wants to test the patient for myocardial infarction in order to rule out the disease as a possible reason for the patient's illness.

76.

B. "UTI" is a term that means "urinary tract infection."

77.

C. Pathy is the usual suffix used to identify a condition. For example, cardiomyopathy is the disease of the myocardium or the heart muscle.

78.

D. "s.l" is a route of administration that is given sublingually or under the tongue.

79.

A. "GERD" means gastroesophageal reflux disease.

80.

C. "Cata" has the meaning of breakdown as in catabolism such as the breakdown of substances into energy.

81.

C. Fluoxetine is the generic name for PROZAC. Therefore, you can infer that filgrastim is a generic name and its corresponding brand name is NEUPOGEN.

82.

A. MAALOX comes in a liquid form called a suspension. Suspensions are when finely divided and nondissolved drugs are dispersed in liquid vehicles. This causes sedimentation of the drugs to the bottom of the bottle; therefore, all suspensions require the user to shake the bottle well before use.

83.

B. The bevel is the term given for the small, oval-shaped opening in a needle through which fluid is drawn.

84.

B. "Erythro" means redness and the word erythrocyte means red blood cell.

85.

C. D12.5 is a bag that does not come premixed from the manufacturer. The other three do come premixed. The 3%NS is a hyperosmotic saline solution.

86.

D. ALEVE is the only medication of the four listed that is an OTC. It is a pain reliever.

87.

D. "MDI" means metered-dose inhaler. It is found on orders where the doctor has written for the use of an inhaler, like albuterol or ipratropium. The term means that each dose a patient takes in has an accurate measure of a specific amount of drug.

88.

B. The term used to denote blood cells that are irregularly shaped is sickle cell. In this case, the cells are bent and twisted to look like a sickle.

89.

A. "DNA" means deoxyribonucleic acid and is the genetic code of the human body.

90.

A. "DT" stands for delirium tremens.

91.

A. Delirium, in general, is an altered state of consciousness with agitation, hyperactivity, and disorientation. Tremens is a specific type of delirium brought about by alcohol withdrawal after a sustained period of intoxication.

92.

D. "COPD" stands for chronic obstructive pulmonary disease.

93.

D. a.u. stands for each ear.

94.

B. "Brady" means slow. For bradycardia, the word means slow heart rate or heartbeat.

95.

C. "CNS" means central nervous system.

96.

A. "Neuro" refers to the nerves of the body, like the word neurolysis, which is the destruction of the nervous tissue.

97.

C. HCO_3 represents the chemical bicarbonate, as in sodium bicarbonate.

98.

B. Mg represents magnesium. It has affects on the heart and its ability to pump blood in the human body.

99.

C. PLETAL is an antiplatelet drug used to allow the blood to flow more smoothly in the body.

100.

A. Ca represents the chemical calcium. Calcium, along with magnesium and potassium, has profound effects on the heart.

101.

C. "algia" and "dynia" refer to symptoms associated with pain.

102.

B. The horizontal flow hood is the type of hood used to prepare those IV admixtures that are not chemo agents. The horizontal flow allows particles and bacteria to dissipate away from the manipulation area, keeping the final product sterile.

103.

B. "oma" usually denotes a tumor, like in carcinoma or melanoma.

104.

D. Na represents sodium.

105.

C. "mg/kg/dose" stands for milligram per kilogram per dose. This is used to designate dosing of a drug based on the patient's weight. For each kilogram of weight, a patient must get a certain amount of milligram per dose.

106.

D. "malacia" refers to the softening or loss of consistency of any of the organs or tissues.

107.

C. K represents potassium, as in KCl. Potassium is important to regulation of heart rate but a higher than normal level could also lead to arrythmias of the heart.

108.

D. "NSAIDs" refers to the class of agents called non-steroidal anti-inflammatory drugs.

109.

B. Li represents lithium. Lithium was one of the first agents used to treat psychosis or conditions affecting the mental capacity of an individual.

110.

B. The suffix "itis" commonly refers to an inflammation of some sort, like arthritis.

111.

A. "OTC" means over the counter, medication that does not require a physician's order to dispense and use.

112.

A. "PCA" stands for patient-controlled analgesia. In this case, the patient was allowed to determine how much he or she gets, within limits, of a pain control medication.

113.

D. "Rhin" refers to the nose.

114.

B. SERAX is the only drug of the four listed that belongs in the benzodiazepine class.

115.

D. The prefix "litho" has the meaning of calcification, as in lithotripsy, which means crushing of a stone in the renal pelvix or bladder.

116.

B. "Cere" refers to the brain, as in cerebellum.

117.

C. "PCN" stands for the drug penicillin.

118.

C. The term LMWH stands for low molecular weight heparin. This refers to drugs like LOVENOX.

119.

D. Chondrodynia means pain in the cartilage. "Chondro" means cartilage.

120.

D. "PUD" means peptic ulcer disease.

121.

B. Homeostasis is a term that refers to the normal functioning of the human body, while hemostasis refers to properties of vasoconstriction.

122.

B. Mastodynia refers to pain in the breast area.

123.

A. NTG is a term referring to the drug nitroglycerin.

124.

A. "RA" stands for the disease rheumatoid arthritis.

125.

B. "Gloss" refers to the tongue and glossitis means inflammation of the tongue.

126.

A. # is usually followed by a number for the quantity to dispense.

127.

D. Renal impact refers to effects a drug has on the kidney.

128.

B. "XL" means that the medication is made in an extended release formulation.

129.

B. "SOB" refers to shortness of breath.

130.

B. Both terms refer to the blood. Hyperemia means having a presence of a high amount of blood in an organ. Hemapoiesis means producing red blood cells.

131.

D. NB is a designation you would not find on a presciption order. The term has a few meanings and one of them is newborn.

132.

C. CRNA stands for certified registered nurse anesthetist. They help and support the anesthesiologist during surgeries but are not allowed to prescribe medications.

133.

D. "Gastr" refers to the stomach. Gastritis means inflammation of the stomach.

134.

C. "SSRI" refers to selective serotonin reuptake inhibitor. It designates a class of drugs used to treat depression.

135.

A. DOSS or DSS is a medication used to treat constipation since it is a laxative. The medication term is short for docustate sodium.

136.

D. "Cardium" refers to the heart. Pericardium means the outer covering around the heart.

137.

B. Cardiac drugs affect the heart.

138.

B. "Tachy" means accelerated or fast. Tachycardia means fast heartbeat or heart rate.

139.

D. "TCA" means tricyclic antidepressants. It was one of the first classes of drugs used to treat depression.

140.

C. Heparin is the only one of the four that would have "units" designated after the strength.

141.

D. The prefix "semi" means partial.

142.

A. JCAHO is a nongovernmental body that accredits hospitals in general and other health care facilities. The Joint Commission on Accreditation of Health-care Organizations usually reviews hospitals every 3 years.

143.

B. "Peri" refers to around or surrounding. Pericarditis means inflammation of the pericardium, which is the area surrounding the heart.

144.

A. "TCN" stands for the drug tetracycline.

145.

B. Glycosuria means finding sugar in the urine.

146.

A. First, you must know that PTCA means percutaneous transluminal coronary angioplasty. Abciximab is a drug used during procedures to prevent ischemic complications within 12 hours after the procedure.

147.

A. Dyspnea means having difficulty in breathing.

148.

D. C means 100 in Roman numerals and c means "with" or "in addition to."

149.

D. Intracranially means occurring within the skull since "cran" means skull and "intra" means within.

150.

A. VICODIN is a controlled drug. It is important to verify that the DEA number of the doctor on the prescription is valid in order to deter any fraudulent prescription or actions.

151.

D. The normal unit of measurement used for BSA is m^2. BSA is the acronym for Body Surface Area.

152.

C. b.i.d. means, in any order, twice a day.

153.

D. Before you make any antineoplastic agent, a.k.a. chemo drug, you should wear double gloves and a gown buttoned in the back for your own protection.

154.

C. A target for a pharmacodynamic drug is a receptor, whether it be the heart or kidney. A receptor is a site with a configuration that resembles the chemical structure of a drug. This allows it to "hook on" and act in the proper fashion.

155.

D. "qhs" means getting it at bedtime or at night. So since bedtime is once a day, a "qd" amount of "qhs" would be just one.

156.

C. ERYTHROCIN does not normally require routine blood levels. The other three must have blood levels due to possibility of toxicity if overdosed.

157.

C. *MedWatch* is a program that keeps track of adverse events. The monitoring of adverse events that a drug can produce is important because it allows a post-marketing study of a drug and helps to determine if a drug has adverse effects that could be severe and life-threatening. This could lead to a drug being pulled from the market in an event that is serious enough to be fatal in humans.

4 Dispensing Process and Information Resources

chapter objectives

Students will demonstrate knowledge in:

➤ Understanding and interpreting prescriptions and medication orders

➤ The area of proper labeling of medications in the process of dispensing

➤ Product preparation in the dispensing process

➤ Areas requiring special activities with regard to dispensing

➤ Safe medication practices

➤ Common ailments and associated drug treatments

➤ The area of pharmacokinetics to a certain extent

DIRECTIONS Each of the questions or incomplete statements below is followed by suggested answers or completions. Select the **one answer** that is best in each case.

1. What steps should be taken when the prescriber's DEA number is missing from a prescription for a controlled substance?
   A. Leave it blank.
   B. Call the prescriber's office for verification and the DEA number.
   C. Enter a universal DEA number.
   D. Call the DEA for the prescriber's number.

2. What is meant by "ibuprofen 400 mg. PO QID c food stat"?
   A. Give 400 mg of ibuprofen with meals every day immediately.
   B. Give 400 mg of ibuprofen with food four times a day and provide a status.
   C. Give ibuprofen 400 mg with food every 4 hours.
   D. Give 400 mg of ibuprofen orally with food four times a day starting immediately.

3. Use of abbreviations on a prescription label is limited to which of the following?
   A. Use abbreviations for commonly used words.
   B. Use abbreviations to conserve space on the label.
   C. Never use abbreviations.
   D. Use abbreviations to complete a heavy prescription workload in a timely manner.

4. Why is it important to have the full name of the patient on the prescription?
   A. The drug charge will go to the right party.
   B. The law requires the full name.
   C. This ensures the right drug will be dispensed to the right patient.
   D. It is necessary for insurance purposes.

5. What is the meaning of "D/C ciprofloxacin start cephalexin 500 mg. PO QID × 14 D"?

   A. Stop ciprofloxacin and start cephalexin at 500 mg by mouth four times a day for 14 doses.
   B. Stop ciprofloxacin and start cephalexin 500 mg every 6 hours for 14 days.
   C. Discontinue ciprofloxacin. Start cephalexin 500 mg orally three times a day for 14 doses.
   D. Discontinue the ciprofloxacin. Start cephalexin 500 mg orally four times a day for 14 days.

6. What is the script?
   A. the prescription
   B. the counseling format
   C. the writing on the prescription blank
   D. the original handwritten order

7. What does a traditional prescription order provide?
   A. pricing
   B. the information needed to fill the medication order accurately
   C. third-party payer requirements
   D. a method to communicate the patient's illness

8. "MSO_4 0.002g IV push q2° prn for breakthrough pain for 9 h only" means what?
   A. Give 0.002g of magnesium sulfate through an intravenous push for breakthrough pain for only 9 hours.
   B. Give manganese sulfate 2 mg, pushing it in an intravenous fluid volume running every 2 hours for breakthrough pain for the next 9 hours.
   C. Give 2 mg of morphine sulfate through an intravenous push every 2 hours when needed for breakthrough pain for up to 9 hours only.
   D. none of the above

9. The term CE in pharmacy stands for
   A. certified employee
   B. counting extra
   C. compounding extemporaneously
   D. continuing education

10. Which of the following auxiliary labels is appropriate for a prescription containing acetaminophen and codeine?
    A. May cause photosensitivity.
    B. Drink plenty of fluids.
    C. May cause drowsiness.
    D. Finish all this medication unless otherwise directed by prescriber.

11. What does "alprazolam 0.25 mg. PO × 1 stat" mean?
    A. Give alprazolam 25 mg orally—provide one-time status.
    B. Give alprazolam 0.25 mg tablet orally one-time immediately.
    C. Give alprazolam 0.25 mg starting at 1:00 P.M.
    D. Give alprazolam 0.25 mg by mouth with first dose starting now.

12. Which strip label is very important to affix to all antibiotic prescriptions?
    A. May cause discoloration of urine or feces.
    B. Take with food or milk.
    C. Finish all this medication unless otherwise directed by prescriber.
    D. This drug may impair the ability to drive or operate machinery.

13. What steps should you take when in doubt about the directions on a prescription?
    A. Use "as directed" for the directions.
    B. Tell the patient to check with their doctor.
    C. Call the doctor's office for verification of drug and clarification of directions.
    D. Do the best interpretation possible.

14. What does "D/C p.o. hydroxyzine. Give hydroxyzine 25 mg. IM q3–4h c meperidine IV 75 mg. PRN pain" mean?
    A. Discontinue the oral hydroxyzine. Give hydroxyzine 25 mg intramuscularly every 3–4 hours with meperidine 75 mg intravenously as needed for pain.
    B. Stop the rectal hydroxyzine and give 25 mg of hydroxyzine intramuscularly every 3 or 4 hours with meperidine 75 mg when needed for pain.
    C. Stop hydroxyzine by mouth. Give 25 mg of it intramuscularly over 3 to 4 hours with 75 mg of meperidine as needed.
    D. Discontinue the oral hydroxyzine. Give 25 mg of hydroxyzine in a muscle every 3 or 4 hours with meperidine #4 in 75 mg doses as needed for pain.

15. What is the best way to provide additional special instructions to the patient that he or she will not forget?
    A. Affix a strip or auxiliary label on the container.
    B. Provide the patient with the reference page number.
    C. Tell the patient.
    D. All instructions must be typed on the label affixed to the container.

16. What is missing or incorrect from the following: "Zantac 150mg po for 7 days"?
    A. The route is incorrect.
    B. The strength does not exist for that drug.
    C. The frequency is missing.
    D. There is nothing wrong with it.

17. How would you translate "Famotidine susp. 20 mg. pGT q. d."?
    A. famotidine sisps 20 mg after gastric treatment every day
    B. famotidine suspension 20 mg per drop every day

C. famotidine suspension 20 mg per gastric tube every day

D. famotidine susceptibility 20 mg per gastric test every day

18. Of the following, which one would make filling a prescription difficult if it were missing?
    A. number of refills
    B. patient's age
    C. generic name of the drug
    D. amount to be taken

19. Which is the usual direction for administering p.o. tablets?
    A. insert
    B. apply
    C. take
    D. place

20. How would you explain the directions for Propoxyphene-N-100,1 PO q4–6° prn HA?
    A. Take a tablet every 4 hours if needed for headache. Take one every 6 hours if not severe.
    B. Take one tablet orally every 4 to 6 hours when needed for headache.
    C. Take one tablet by mouth every 4–6 hours for hypertensive activity.
    D. Take one tablet every 4 or 6 hours when needed for headache.

21. Which of the following answers best describes what the prescription sig should contain?
    A. the name of the drug, how to take the drug, and the time
    B. the number of units, dosage form, frequency or specific time, and administration method

C. the administration route, the number of units, the frequency, and the side effects

D. the administration route, the frequency, the number of units, and the price

22. Which is the best way to describe in the directions the way to use an external ointment?
    A. apply
    B. insert
    C. instill
    D. take

23. What is the best way to describe the method of using a suppository?
    A. apply
    B. take
    C. instill
    D. insert

24. What are the directions for phenytoin 400 mg. p.o. stat, repeat in 4 hours, then 100 mg. PO q8h? (NOTE: Use phenytoin 100 mg. capsules)
    A. Take four capsules now and again in 4 hours. Then take 100 mg every 8 hours.
    B. Take four capsules by mouth at once and in 4 hours, then take one capsule by mouth every 8 hours.
    C. Take 400 mg now, four capsules in 4 hours, and 100 mg orally every 8 hours.
    D. Take eight capsules within 4 hours and follow with one capsule every 8 hours thereafter.

25. How many ccs are in a tuberculin syringe?
    A. 10 cc
    B. 5 cc
    C. 3 cc
    D. 1 cc

26. Which is the best way to describe in the directions the way to use eyedrops?
    A. apply
    B. insert
    C. instill
    D. take

27. If a patient asks you a medically related question, you should
    A. answer it to the best of your knowledge
    B. call the pharmacist over to talk to the patient
    C. ignore them since it is beyond your job description
    D. tell them that they should consult a doctor

28. Which of the following is the best direction to a patient for diphenhydramine 50 mg. p.o. q6h prn pruritis?
    A. Take one capsule by mouth every 6 hours when needed for itching.
    B. Take one pill every 6 hours as needed for sleeping problems.
    C. Take one every 6 hours for insomnia.
    D. Take one capsule orally every 6 hours when needed.

29. Which of the following routes of administration provides the fastest action?
    A. subq
    B. IM
    C. IV
    D. SL

30. Which drug of the following listed comes in tablet and oral inhalation forms?
    A. ipratropium
    B. albuterol
    C. salmeterol
    D. beclomethasone

31. In addition to vials and ovals, other containers to package drugs for ambulatory patients include which of the following?
    A. ointment jars
    B. plastic bags
    C. dropper bottles
    D. answers A and C

32. ROBITUSSIN DAC contains three ingredients, where two are guaifenesin and codeine. What is the third?
    A. phenylephrine
    B. dextromethorphan
    C. pseudoephedrine
    D. promethazine

33. What does it mean to give a drug p.c.?
    A. through a personal catheter
    B. as a prepaid claim
    C. after meals
    D. before meals

34. The abbreviation PPD stands for purified protein derivative. Which of the following drug is PPD associated with?
    A. Diphtheria-tetanus
    B. Tuberculin
    C. Antivenin
    D. Heparin

35. The label on a bulk bottle of a medication is important because it contains vital information such as what?
    A. the drug name
    B. the drug strength
    C. the expiration date of the drug
    D. all of the above

36. If there is **suspected** diversion of narcotics, which of the following must you file a report to?
    A. ASHP
    B. Office of State Board of Pharmacy

C. DEA

D. both B and C

37. What should you do in the event of doubtful directions?

A. Ask the patient.

B. Leave it up to the pharmacist to check you.

C. Clarify the directions before filling any prescription order.

D. Make your best guess.

38. What are the directions for $MgSO_4$ 2 Gm. IV in 100 cc. NS over 1°?

A. magnesium sulfate 2 grams intravenously in 100 cc of normal saline over 1 hour

B. morphine sulfate 2 grams intravenously in 100 cc normal sulfate over 1 hour

C. manganese sulfate 2 Gm intravenously in 100 cc of normal saline over 1 hour

D. magnesium sulfate 2 milligrams in 100 cc of Ringer's solution over 1 hour

39. In a weight-to-volume product of dextrose 50%, which of the following best describes the concentration of dextrose?

A. The product is half dextrose.

B. 50 mg of dextrose in 100 ml of water

C. 50 Gm of dextrose in 100 ml of water

D. 50 mg of dextrose in 50 cc of water

40. Never dispense _____.

A. ointments with an "External use only" label

B. a prescription with a red-bordered label

C. capsules in a plastic vial

D. guesswork

41. A technician can do all the following except

A. count pills

B. counsel patients on new medications

C. stock narcotics on the shelves

D. pull the medication from the shelves

42. In the hospital setting when reviewing a physician's order for drugs, in addition to the medications, strength, and frequency for use, what else is essential to review to ensure the safety and well-being of a patient?

A. nonpharmaceutical services performed

B. legibility of the nurse's and doctor's signatures

C. date of admission

D. allergies or sensitivities to drugs and foods

43. What essential information should be on a repackaged medication dispensed to a hospitalized patient?

A. No information additional to the labeled information on the drug is necessary.

B. patient's name, patient's room number and bed number, and date

C. Only the name and strength of the drug is essential.

D. Only the room and bed numbers are needed.

44. Why are auxillary strips necessary?

A. They provide additional room for information that cannot be typed on the primary label.

B. These labels are necessary to cover an open area on the container.

C. They provide additional information about using or taking the medication properly.

D. Strip labels are required by law.

45. When do you need the pharmacist and pharmacy technician's initials on the prescription?

A. when the drug is filled by the technician and checked by the pharmacist

B. during work hours to acknowledge the presence of staff

C. The pharmacist's and technician's initials are unnecessary.

D. The initials are needed for controlled drug substances only.

46. In the hospital setting, the MAR stands for
    A. maximum attendance requirement
    B. medication activity report
    C. medium acceptable record
    D. medication administration record

47. Of the following, which drug is considered the first-line agent for any cardiac arrest or code blue in the hospital setting?
    A. calcium chloride
    B. adenosine
    C. sodium bicarb
    D. epinephrine

48. Phosphate mixed with this other chemical can cause an unwanted precipitation in IV bags.
    A. potassium
    B. magnesium
    C. calcium
    D. selenium

49. What are the directions for meperidine in "Meperidine 50 mg. IM q 4h prn pain"?
    A. 50 mg every 4 minutes as needed for pain
    B. 50 mg intermittently in 4 hours when needed for pain
    C. 50 mg intramuscularly every 4 hours as needed for pain
    D. 50 mg injected every 4 hours as needed for pain

50. What is another way of writing twice daily after meals?
    A. BID pc
    B. B × D pc
    C. 2 xid pc
    D. BID ac

51. How would you start the directions for a prescription for nose drops?
    A. take

B. instill
C. apply
D. insert

52. When you withdraw medication from an ampule, what must you use that you don't need to use for vials?
    A. filter needle
    B. gloves
    C. a sterile air flow hood
    D. aseptic technique

53. A prescription label must contain information that includes
    A. the prescriber's name, the prescriber's office staff who called in the refill, and the date of the next refill
    B. the patient's address, the patient's gender, the patient's age, and the patient's nationality
    C. the payer's social security number, the insurance company name, the remaining deductible, and the co-insurance
    D. the prescription number, the patient's full name, directions for taking the medication, the prescriber's name, the date, and the name of the drug

54. Why is knowing the age of the patient important?
    A. The age may determine what dosage form should be used.
    B. The age may indicate if the dosage is appropriate.
    C. Age is never important.
    D. answers A and B

55. A prescription for a controlled substance must contain what required elements?
    A. the practitioner's office address
    B. the practitioner's DEA number
    C. the practitioner's signature
    D. all of the above

56. If no entry is made in the refills box, should you refill the drug?
    A. yes
    B. no
    C. maybe
    D. depends on the pharmacy policy

57. What are some indications that there has been tampering with the prescription?
    A. The written quantity of drug is smudged.
    B. The ink color or shade varies.
    C. The first name of the patient has been added where the prescriber wrote only the surname.
    D. answers A and B

58. What are some important things to look for on the prescription blank?
    A. The name of the patient is clear and correct.
    B. The drug can be substituted therapeutically.
    C. The drug name and quantity are written clearly.
    D. answers A and C

59. When is a prescriber's DEA number used?
    A. The DEA number is used if the drug is part of the Drug Evaluation Act.
    B. The DEA number is an arbitrary number that has little use in pharmacy practice.
    C. The DEA number is used to indicate the prescriber is a medical doctor and not an osteopath.
    D. The DEA number is required when the prescriber writes a prescription for a controlled substance.

60. The model prescription order contains which of the following elements?
    A. patient's name and address
    B. drug name, strength, and form

    C. quantity of the drug to be dispensed
    D. all of the above

61. What should be the primary concern of the pharmacy technician?
    A. The pharmacy is well-stocked at all times.
    B. The work area is clean.
    C. The safety and well-being of the patient is the primary concern.
    D. All records are maintained appropriately.

62. When weighing ingredients for compounding by using a torsion balance, what instrument do you use to pick up the individual weights?
    A. fingers
    B. weighing paper
    C. small tweezer
    D. weights aren't needed with torsion balance

63. What types of practitioners can write prescriptions for legend drugs?
    A. physicians, osteopaths, dentists, veterinarians
    B. doctors of education, doctors of philosophy
    C. doctors of jurisprudence, psychologists, doctors of pharmacy
    D. none of the above

64. What is the purpose of having distilled water in the dispensing area?
    A. Distilled water is used to reconstitute medications requiring the addition of water.
    B. Distilled water is used for cleaning sinks and compounding countertops.
    C. Distilled water used to bathe patients with contagious diseases is supplied by the pharmacy.
    D. all of the above

65. Distributive pharmacy consists of a prescription order-processing activity and a
medication product-preparation function.
Which of the following functions does the
pharmacy technician perform during the
preparation phase?
    A. places orders for the required medica-
tions
    B. obtains patient health information
    C. retrieves the medication
    D. helps patrons with OTC needs

66. Which is not a drug delivery system?
    A. metered-dose inhaler (MDI)
    B. transdermal patch
    C. magnetic carrier transport
    D. ophthalmic drops

67. There may be evidence that any medication
that interacts with erythromycin, ketaconazole, or itraconazole may also interact with
which of the following fruit juices?
    A. orange
    B. apple
    C. grapefruit
    D. cranberry

68. Which term best describes an interaction in
which one drug enhances the effect of another medication?
    A. antagonistic drug interaction
    B. synergistic drug interaction
    C. pharmacokinetic drug interaction
    D. none of the above

69. What technique is used to ease the withdrawal of a solution from a vial?
    A. Place an additional hole in the di-
aphragm next to the transfer site.
    B. Always make the withdrawal of solution
in at least two steps.

C. Inject a volume of air equal to the volume of solution for withdrawal into the
vial before withdrawal.
    D. Shake vial immediately prior to with-
drawing the solution.

70. Which term best describes an interaction in
which one drug cancels out the effect of another medication?
    A. synergistic drug interaction
    B. additive drug interaction
    C. antagonistic drug interaction
    D. none of the above

71. Acetaminophen products containing
codeine have the potential to cause what
side effect?
    A. blurred vision
    B. drowsiness
    C. cough
    D. diarrhea

72. When compounding a product in a horizontal air flow hood, how far in from the front
of the hood should you be working?
    A. 10 inches
    B. 5 inches
    C. doesn't matter
    D. 6 inches

73. Since acetaminophen or a compound containing acetaminophen is metabolized in the
liver, monitor closely if the patient is taking
which of the following drug group(s)?
    A. alcohol
    B. tuberculosis drugs
    C. anticonvulsants
    D. all of the above

74. A primary reason why patients do not comply with the directions for taking medications is which of the following?
    A. The medication is not aesthetically
pleasing.

B. A friend or family member tells the patient not to take it.

C. The patient does not understand the directions.

D. The patient takes the medication as he or she wants.

75. Hospital pharmacy practice deals primarily with what type of patient?

A. ambulatory

B. institutionalized

C. adult day care

D. clinic

76. What is characteristic of a solution?

A. Solutions have specific colors.

B. Solutes are suspended in a solvent.

C. All solutes are dissolved in the solvent.

D. Solutes in solution must have a specific surface area.

77. What is characteristic of a suspension?

A. Solutes are dissolved in a thick solvent.

B. All suspensions must be refrigerated.

C. Suspension expiration dates are longer than those for solutions.

D. Solutes are suspended in the solvent.

78. Community pharmacy practice deals primarily with what type of patient?

A. institutionalized

B. inpatient

C. ambulatory

D. home infusion

79. What is the purpose of a buffer used in admixtures?

A. It keeps pH from changing with the addition of acids or bases to the mixture.

B. It prevents the drug from deteriorating the stomach lining.

C. It extends the period of activity for the active ingredient.

D. It ensures sterility of the mixture.

80. Which of the following drugs works therapeutically by impacting on leukotrienes?

A. zileuton

B. zafirlukast

C. zalcitabine

D. answers A and B

81. What is the most important thing to remember when preparing IV admixtures?

A. Always use aseptic technique.

B. Never forget to initial the label.

C. Always run electrolytes separately into the evacuated container.

D. Never use a plastic container when glass is available.

82. Why must you be especially careful of selling to a diabetic patient a drug in a syrup vehicle?

A. Syrup preparations may contain a high concentration of sugar.

B. The sodium content enhances the effect of oral hypoglycemic agents.

C. The alcohol content tends to decrease blood sugar.

D. none of the above

83. Which of the following reasons best supports levigation in compounding a suspension?

A. It decreases surface area.

B. It enhances the viscosity of the preparation.

C. It enhances the palatability of the preparation.

D. It reduces particle size.

84. What is the major source of contamination in an IV admixture program?

A. personnel

B. materials and equipment

C. the environment

D. all of the above

85. Which of the following capsule sizes has the largest capacity?

    A. 000
    B. 1
    C. 4
    D. 5

86. Which of the following drug vehicles does not contain alcohol?

    A. elixir
    B. fluid extracts
    C. syrup
    D. tinctures

87. What is the purpose of using aseptic technique to prepare IV admixtures?

    A. to comply with JCAHO rules
    B. to comply with Boards of Pharmacy
    C. to prevents contamination of the final product
    D. to protect yourself from contact with toxic drugs

88. What method best accomplishes blending a powder into a cream base?

    A. sifting
    B. shaking
    C. levigation
    D. titrating

89. Which of the following is the most commonly used paper for weighing drugs on a balance?

    A. glassine
    B. parchment
    C. bond
    D. waxed

90. How long will 1L of an IV last that is running at 4.2 ml/minute?

    A. nearly 4 hours
    B. nearly 238 hours
    C. nearly 24 hours
    D. nearly 6 hours

91. Which of the following answers best describes the pharmacokinetics of a drug?

    A. ionization, mediation, and diffusion
    B. bioavailability, ionization, and transport
    C. absorption, distribution, and elimination
    D. polarity, molecular weight, and receptor affinity

92. Which are the primary organs involved in drug elimination?

    A. liver and kidney
    B. lungs
    C. spleen and gall bladder
    D. stomach and intestines

93. An order for an IV admixture includes the addition of 4,000 units of heparin. What volume from the 10,000u/ml vial will provide 4,000 units?

    A. 0.5 ml
    B. 0.6 ml
    C. 0.04 ml
    D. 0.4 ml

94. What organ performs renal drug elimination?

    A. skin
    B. kidney
    C. intestine
    D. liver

95. What organ performs hepatic drug biotransformations?

    A. kidney
    B. spleen
    C. liver
    D. pancreas

96. What are some of the components of a traditional TPN?

    A. amino acids, lactated ringers, vitamins
    B. amino acids, dextrose, electrolytes, vitamins

C. amino acids, normal saline, electrolytes

D. amino acids, sterile water, lipids, electrolytes

97. What organ has responsibility for producing insulin?

    A. pancreas

    B. liver

    C. kidney

    D. adrenals

98. The term bioavailability best refers to which one of the following answers?

    A. the amount of drug detoxified in the liver

    B. the amount of drug remaining for therapeutic effect after elimination from the kidneys

    C. the rate and amount of therapeutically active drug that reaches systemic circulation

    D. the balance between the physical and chemical properties of a drug and the net therapeutic effect that remains

99. What is another name for the "fat" used in TPN or alone as an IV?

    A. triglycerides

    B. lipids

    C. cholesterols

    D. lipoproteins

100. For any type of TPN, what is the maximum amount of time it is allowed to be hung without changing a new bag?

    A. 10 hours

    B. 18 hours

    C. 20 hours

    D. 24 hours

101. The movement of drug molecules across a cell membrane from a region of high drug concentration to a region of low drug concentration is best known by which of the following answers?

    A. passive diffusion

    B. active transport

    C. bioavailability

    D. zero-order absorption

102. What should be done before clamping and cutting the transfer set attached to the finished IV product?

    A. Expel air from the flexible bag.

    B. Visually examine the final product for particles.

    C. Weigh the final product.

    D. Affix the label.

103. CLARITIN is usually given for what condition?

    A. infection

    B. allergies

    C. hypertension

    D. arthritis

104. What condition is most likely to use the HMG-CoA reductase inhibitor class of drugs?

    A. asthma

    B. hyperlipidemia

    C. hypertension

    D. diabetes

105. If a patient needs a proton pump inhibitor to be given IV, which one would you choose?

    A. PRILOSEC

    B. ACIPHEX

    C. PROTONIX

    D. PREVACID

106. What condition is most likely associated with leukotrienes?

    A. AIDS

    B. diabetes

    C. asthma

    D. depression

107. What component of a dosage form elicits the pharmacologic action?
    A. lubricant
    B. excipient
    C. binder
    D. active ingredient

108. Which of the following controlled substances would commonly be used in surgery?
    A. VICODIN
    B. VERSED
    C. VALIUM
    D. TYLENOL #3

109. Why are there various types of dosage forms?
    A. to accommodate different ages and conditions of patients
    B. to make the medication palatable
    C. to permit maximum drug availability and absorption
    D. all of the above

110. What is/are an example(s) of solid dosage forms?
    A. suspensions
    B. capsules
    C. lotions
    D. answers A and C

111. If you are compounding in a laminar flow hood, what is recommended that you do?
    A. Go in and out of the hood whenever you need to.
    B. You are allowed to talk in the hood about subjects relating to your job.
    C. Wash your hands with an approved solution each time you leave and reenter the hood.
    D. You may keep rings on your hands, but not watches.

112. Typical topical dosage forms include which of the following?
    A. ointments
    B. creams
    C. transdermal patches
    D. all of the above

113. What could you expect a patient taking drugs for hypertension to be doing?
    A. maintaining a low-salt diet
    B. maintaining a low-carbohydrate diet
    C. maintaining a low-protein diet
    D. maintaining a "force-fluids" diet

114. Who traditionally decides which drugs will be part of the formulary?
    A. hospital upper management
    B. pharmacy and Nursing Workgroup
    C. the Pharmacy and Therapueutics Committee
    D. the Board of Pharmacy

115. Which triple-drug therapy is used to treat ulcers caused by *Helicobacter pylori*?
    A. omeprazole-amoxicillin-clarithromycin
    B. PEPTO-BISMOL-metronidazole-tetracycline or amoxicillin
    C. omeprazole-metronidazole-clarithromycin
    D. all of the above

116. Which directions should require clarification?
    A. Take medication three times a day.
    B. Ut. dict. or take medication as directed.
    C. Take medication every day.
    D. Take medication at bedtime.

117. In general, what is a formulary?
    A. formulas used for compounding
    B. a carefully selected, limited list of drugs

C. drugs reimbursed by insurance companies

D. a list of drugs used with disease management systems

118. What is a prevalent reason for medication errors?
A. wrong patient
B. wrong address
C. poor legibility
D. no refills listed

119. The extended release or nonimmediate release form of CARDIZEM has what abbreviation?
A. XL
B. CD
C. SR
D. ER

120. Which of the following elements helps to determine what drugs are included in a formulary?
A. the safety of the drug
B. the margin of potential drug errors
C. control of drug purchasing costs
D. all of the above

121. Factors contributing to dispensing errors include
A. excessive workload
B. excessive interruptions
C. inadequate training
D. all of the above

122. Amino acids in TPN provides a source of nitrogen for
A. protein anabolism
B. protein metabolism
C. calories
D. energy anabolism

123. What contains a large percentage of solid material and are thicker and stiffer than ointments?

A. tinctures
B. paste
C. powder
D. liniments

124. Another reference to osteoarthritis may include which of the following?
A. inflammation of the arterioles
B. degenerative joint disease
C. inflamed adrenal glands
D. degenerative lung flexibility

125. Which of the following drugs would be expected as part of the pharmaceutical management for hemorrhoids?
A. ibuprofen
B. aminucuproic acid
C. carisoprodol
D. hydrocortisone

126. The desired range for room temperature would be
A. 8–15°C
B. 2–8°C
C. 15–30°C
D. 20–40°C

127. Nonpharmaceutical management to treat chronic obstructive pulmonary disease should include which of the following?
A. no smoking
B. bland diet
C. heating pad
D. orthotics

128. How would you characterize the organ impacted by restricted pulmonary air flow?
A. heart
B. kidneys
C. lungs
D. liver

129. Nonpharmaceutical management to treat depression may include which of the following?
    A. UV therapy
    B. reclusion
    C. light therapy
    D. PT

130. Nonpharmaceutical management to treat fever should include which of the following?
    A. warm alcohol bath
    B. cool compresses
    C. high bulk diet
    D. pressed cucumber rub

131. Which of the following drugs would be expected as part of the pharmaceutical management for diarrhea?
    A. loperamide
    B. nizatidine
    C. phenytoin
    D. colchicine

132. The class of drugs known as "triptans" is used for which of the following conditions?
    A. obesity
    B. nausea/vomiting
    C. migraine headaches
    D. vertigo

133. Which of the following drug types or drug classes is expected to appear in a pharmaceutical management regimen for constipation?
    A. laxatives
    B. antiemetics
    C. antinauseants
    D. expectorants

134. Nonpharmaceutical management to treat digestive tract ulcers should include which of the following?
    A. exercise program
    B. diet free from irritating foods
    C. psychotherapy
    D. low-sodium diet

135. Which of the following drugs would be expected as part of the pharmaceutical management for epilepsy?
    A. lovastatin
    B. paclitaxol
    C. allopurinol
    D. phenytoin

136. Which of the following would be considered an ophthalmic agent?
    A. lansoprazole
    B. betamethasone
    C. promethazine
    D. cyclopentolate

137. Which of the following drugs would be expected as part of the pharmaceutical management for asthma?
    A. terazosin
    B. thioridazine
    C. terconazole
    D. theophylline

138. Of the drugs listed, which one is considered a chemo or antineoplastic agent?
    A. ciprofloxacin
    B. carboplatin
    C. celecoxib
    D. carbamazepine

139. Which of the following is NOT a form of iron (ferrous) commonly available in the marketplace?
    A. sulfate
    B. gluconate
    C. hydrochloride
    D. fumarate

140. Another reference to hypertension may include which of the following?
    A. anxiety
    B. high blood pressure
    C. hepatitis
    D. enteritis

141. Nonpharmaceutical management to treat congestive heart failure should include which of the following?
    A. physical therapy
    B. ice packs
    C. low-sodium diet
    D. bland diet

142. Which of the following drug types or drug classes would be expected to appear in a pharmaceutical management regimen for congestive heart failure?
    A. endocrine drugs
    B. diuretics
    C. hormones
    D. antispasmodic drugs

143. Which of the following is considered belonging in the class of drugs called "bisphosphonate"?
    A. pancrelipase
    B. palivizumab
    C. pamidronate
    D. paclitaxel

144. Which of the following drug types or drug classes is expected to appear in a pharmaceutical management regimen for chronic obstructive pulmonary disease?
    A. expectorants
    B. cardiovascular agents
    C. antidiarrheals
    D. antiemetic agents

145. Depression primarily involves which area of human anatomy?

    A. central nervous system
    B. respiratory system
    C. digestive system
    D. female reproductive system

146. What does the word "cirrhosis" refer to?
    A. disease of the pancreas
    B. ringworms
    C. progressive disease of the liver
    D. impairment of the hearing

147. Which of the following drug types or drug classes is expected to appear in a pharmaceutical management regimen for fever?
    A. anti-inflammatories
    B. antineoplastics
    C. antipyretics
    D. anticoagulants

148. If you see drugs like HALDOL and ZYPREXA on a patient's record, what would you conclude?
    A. the patient had severe allergies
    B. the patient had cancer
    C. the patient had ulcers
    D. the patient had a mental illness

149. Which of the following drugs would be expected as part of the pharmaceutical management for constipation?
    A. disopyramide
    B. docusate
    C. dopamide
    D. disulfiram

150. What part of the anatomy is affected by the erosion of the lining of the digestive tract?
    A. esophagus
    B. stomach
    C. intestines
    D. all of the above

151. If a patient is being treated for convulsions, which of the following would likely be prescribed to them?
    A. diltiazem
    B. delestrogen
    C. divalproex
    D. diphenhydramine

152. Which of the following drug types or drug classes is expected to appear in a pharmaceutical management regimen for asthma?
    A. bronchodilators
    B. endocrine agents
    C. hormones
    D. antiemetic agents

153. Nonpharmaceutical management to treat arthritis should include which of the following?
    A. low-sodium diet
    B. specific exercise program
    C. smoking cessation
    D. humidifier

154. A patient is getting ondansetron on a regularly scheduled basis. What can you assume?
    A. the patient is dehydrated
    B. the patient is getting chemotherapy
    C. the patient has an infection
    D. the patient is an alcoholic

155. A patient tells you he just put on his last clonidine patch. How many days later should he get the refill?
    A. 1
    B. 5
    C. 7
    D. 10

156. Which of the following would you NOT give to someone if they had ulcers?
    A. omeprazole
    B. sucralfate
    C. ketorolac
    D. nizatidine

157. Which of the following drugs would be expected as part of the pharmaceutical management for congestive heart failure?
    A. indomethacin
    B. imipramine
    C. ibuprofen
    D. isosorbide

158. Another reference to chronic obstructive pulmonary disease may include which of the following?
    A. chronic bronchitis
    B. constipation
    C. incontinence
    D. thrombosis

159. Which of the following drugs would be expected as part of the pharmaceutical management for chronic obstructive pulmonary disease?
    A. isosorbide
    B. phenytoin
    C. albuterol
    D. colchicine

160. The combination mestranol and norethindrone is a combination that can be found in what class of drugs?
    A. anti-ulcers
    B. hormonal replacement
    C. birth control
    D. antibiotics

161. Which of the following drug types or drug classes is expected to appear in a pharmaceutical management regimen for depression?
    A. cardiovascular agents
    B. psychotherapeutic agents

C. endocrine agents

D. steroids

162. Which of the following drugs would be expected as part of the pharmaceutical management for fever?

A. acetaminophen

B. aspirin

C. meperidine

D. answers A and B

163. Moricizine and flecainide are two drugs in what type of class?

A. antihypertensives

B. antidepressants

C. antiarrythmics

D. antifungals

164. Which organ has a direct involvement on neurological seizure conditions?

A. eyes

B. brain

C. heart

D. intestines

165. Which of the following drug types or drug classes is expected to appear in a pharmaceutical management regimen for stomach ulcers?

A. NSAIDs

B. antacids

C. ACE inhibitors

D. CSF

166. Epilepsy primarily involves which area of human anatomy?

A. central nervous system

B. musculoskeletal system

C. respiratory system

D. digestive system

167. How would you characterize narrowing of the bronchioles in regard to its impact on an organ of the human anatomy?

A. liver

B. kidneys

C. heart

D. lungs

168. How would you characterize the part of anatomy affected by arthritic inflammation?

A. joints

B. skin

C. muscles

D. sinuses

169. Nonpharmaceutical management to treat hemorrhoids should include which of the following?

A. increased dietary fiber

B. warm compresses

C. bland diet

D. orthotics

170. Nonpharmaceutical management to treat hypertension should include which of the following?

A. low-sodium diet

B. low-fat diet

C. exercise program

D. all of the above

171. Which of the following drugs would be expected as part of the pharmaceutical management for lipid disorders?

A. fat emulsions

B. tramadol

C. celecoxib

D. simvastatin

172. A patient may refer to myocardial infarctions by which of the following?

A. heart attack

B. infarct

C. MI

D. all of the above

173. Which of the following drugs would be expected as part of the pharmaceutical management for angina pectoris?
    A. nitroglycerin
    B. nitrofurantoin
    C. nizatidine
    D. nortriptyline

174. All of the following are standard drugs for nausea and vomiting EXCEPT
    A. promethazine
    B. trimethobenzamide
    C. prochlorperazine
    D. trazodone

175. Which of the following drugs could be expected to be part of the pharmaceutical management for atherosclerosis?
    A. loxapine
    B. lorezepam
    C. lovastatin
    D. loperamide

176. Which of the following drugs could be expected as part of the pharmaceutical management for depression?
    A. captopril
    B. diclofenac
    C. sertraline
    D. albuterol

177. The drug tretinoin used topically would possibly be used in which patient population?
    A. teenagers
    B. pediatrics
    C. geriatrics
    D. women

178. Which of the following drug types or drug classes is expected to appear in a pharmaceutical management regimen for diarrhea?
    A. vitamins
    B. electrolyte replacement fluids
    C. antineoplastics
    D. psychotherapeutic agents

179. The drugs listed below are in the same type of antihypertensive class EXCEPT
    A. DIOVAN
    B. COZAAR
    C. MAXZIDE
    D. ATACAND

180. Which of the following drugs could be expected as part of the pharmaceutical management for stomach ulcers?
    A. sucralfate
    B. spironolactone
    C. sulfisoxazole
    D. sulindac

181. Which of the following is a synthetic prostaglandin used to protect the integrity of the stomach lining?
    A. meclizine
    B. lansoprazole
    C. ranitidine
    D. misoprostol

182. Nonpharmaceutical management to treat asthma should include which of the following?
    A. heating pads
    B. massage
    C. removal of irritants from living quarters
    D. high-fiber diet

183. Which of the following drug types or drug classes is expected to appear in a pharmaceutical management regimen for arthritis?
    A. TCA
    B. H_2 antagonist
    C. NSAIDs
    D. protease inhibitors

184. Hemorrhoids primarily involve which part of human anatomy?

    A. diverticulum

    B. hair follicles

    C. skin

    D. veins

185. How would you characterize abnormally high blood pressure in regard to its impact on an organ of the human anatomy?

    A. arteries

    B. blood

    C. intestines

    D. genitals

186. Which of the following laxatives works by increasing the peristaltic contractions of the intestines?

    A. methylcellulose

    B. bisacodyl

    C. docusate sodium

    D. psyllium

187. Myocardial infarctions primarily involve which area of human anatomy?

    A. metabolic system

    B. skeletal system

    C. endocrine system

    D. cardiovascular system

188. Which of the following drug types or drug classes is expected to appear in a pharmaceutical management regimen for angina pectoris?

    A. 5-HT$_3$ receptor agonists

    B. beta-blockers

    C. histamine H$_2$ blockers

    D. proton pump inhibitors

189. Nausea and vomiting primarily involve which areas of human anatomy?

    A. CNS and endocrine system

    B. CNS only

    C. CNS and respiratory system

    D. CNS and digestive system

190. Which of the following drug types or drug classes would you expect to appear in a pharmaceutical management regimen for atherosclerosis?

    A. HMG-CoA reductase inhibitors

    B. NSAIDs

    C. fluoroquinolones

    D. proton pump inhibitors

191. Of the four listed, which one is not an available form of insulin?

    A. 70/30

    B. lispro

    C. glucosamine

    D. glargine

192. Which of the following drugs would be expected as part of the pharmaceutical management for pain?

    A. prochlorperazine

    B. propantheline

    C. propoxyphene napsylate/acetaminophen

    D. propranolol

193. What would you give a patient if they had tinea pedis?

    A. antidepressants

    B. antineoplastics

    C. blood thinners

    D. antifungals

194. Asthma primarily involves which part of the human anatomy?

    A. metabolic system

    B. pulmonary system

    C. endocrine system

    D. digestive system

195. A patient may refer to gastroenteritis by which of the following?
    A. inflamed joints
    B. wheezing
    C. sweats
    D. stomach flu

196. Urinary incontinence is characterized by which of the following?
    A. painful urination
    B. inability to control the bladder
    C. not enough urine output
    D. nocturnal urination

197. Which of the following drugs is used to control urinary incontinence?
    A. TOPROL
    B. ADDERALL
    C. DETROL
    D. ALDOMET

198. Nonpharmaceutical management to treat hypercholesterolemia should include which of the following?
    A. stress management
    B. restricted spice and acidic diet
    C. eliminate saturated fats from diet
    D. psychotherapy

199. Nonpharmaceutical management to treat myocardial infarctions should include which of the following?
    A. smoking cessation
    B. bland diet
    C. restricted exercise
    D. physical therapy

200. How would you characterize restricted coronary blood circulation in regard to its impact on an organ of the human anatomy?
    A. eyes
    B. reproductive system

C. heart and blood vessels
    D. spleen

201. Which of the following drug types or drug classes is expected to appear in a pharmaceutical management regimen for nausea and vomiting?
    A. antiemetics
    B. laxatives
    C. vitamins
    D. psychotherapeutics

202. Which of the following drugs is used to prevent organ rejection in organ transplant cases?
    A. PROVIGIL
    B. PROCARDIA
    C. PROCRIT
    D. PROGRAF

203. Diabetes mellitus primarily involves which area of human anatomy?
    A. respiratory system
    B. skeletal system
    C. reproductive system
    D. endocrine system

204. Which of the following is considered a first-generation antihistamine?
    A. CLARITIN
    B. ZYRTEC
    C. BENADRYL
    D. CLARINEX

205. How would you characterize frequent bowel movements or loose stools in regard to its impact on a body part?
    A. the intestines
    B. the heart
    C. the lungs
    D. the kidneys

206. Gastroenteritis primarily involves which area of human anatomy?

A. endocrine system

B. integumentary system

C. pulmonary system

D. digestive system

207. Which of the following drugs might be expected as part of the pharmaceutical management for gastroenteritis?

A. lomustine

B. loperamide

C. lorazepam

D. loxapine

208. Which of the following drugs can be a part of the pharmaceutical management for hypertension?

A. vecuronium

B. vincristine

C. verapamil

D. valproic acid

209. Lipid disorders primarily involve which area of human anatomy?

A. endocrine system

B. pulmonary system

C. cardiovascular system

D. integumentary system

210. The following are all antibiotics, but one does not belong with the others. Which one is it?

A. LEVAQUIN

B. KEFLEX

C. CIPRO

D. ZAGAM

211. Nonpharmaceutical management to treat angina pectoris should include which of the following?

A. aromatherapy

B. environmental air conditioning

C. orthotics

D. low-fat diet

212. Which of the following drugs could be expected as part of the pharmaceutical management for nausea and vomiting?

A. loperamide

B. docusate

C. prochlorperazine

D. prazosin

213. Nonpharmaceutical management to treat atherosclerosis should include which of the following?

A. low-fat diet

B. weight-management program

C. exercise program

D. all of the above

214. Nonpharmaceutical management to treat diabetes mellitus should include which of the following?

A. heating pads

B. self-monitoring of BP

C. restricted intake of simple sugars

D. necessary orthotics

215. Which of the following drugs would be expected as part of the pharmaceutical management for an uncomplicated headache?

A. amoxapine

B. amiodarone

C. acetaminophen

D. atenolol

216. Which of the following listed is a drug that DOES NOT contain any narcotic product in its formulation?

A. TUSSIONEX

B. RONDEC DM

C. ROBITUSSIN DAC

D. HYCOTUSS

217. Nonpharmaceutical management to treat gastroenteritis should include which of the following?
  A. hot/cold compresses
  B. fetal positioning
  C. electrolyte replacement
  D. raised legs

218. Which other drug belongs in the same class as ACCUZYME OINTMENT?
  A. SANTYL
  B. LIDEX
  C. CLOBETASOL
  D. HALOG

219. Which of the following drug types or drug classes may likely appear in a pharmaceutical management regimen for insomnia?
  A. steroids
  B. histamine H-2 antagonists
  C. antianxiety drugs
  D. antitussive drugs

220. Another reference made to lipid disorders by patients may include which of the following?
  A. runny sinuses
  B. cholesterol
  C. seizures
  D. migraines

221. Which of the following drug types or drug classes is likely to appear in a pharmaceutical management regimen for myocardial infarction?
  A. proton pump inhibitors
  B. colony stimulating factors
  C. antihyperlipidemics
  D. 5 HT-3 receptor agonists

222. Angina pectoris primarily inolves which area of human anatomy?
  A. cardiovascular system
  B. endocrine system
  C. metabolic system
  D. integumentary system

223. Another reference to atherosclerosis may include which of the following?
  A. multiple sclerosis
  B. hardening of the arteries
  C. muscular dystrophy
  D. arterial hypertrophy

224. How would you characterize, relative to an organ, the cause for insufficient metabolism of carbohydrates?
  A. the liver
  B. the pancreas
  C. the kidneys
  D. the lungs

225. Which of the following drugs could be expected as part of the pharmaceutical management for diabetes mellitus?
  A. glyburide
  B. fluoxetine
  C. amlodipine
  D. furosemide

226. The drug amoxicillin is also found in which of the following drugs?
  A. AUGMENTIN
  B. HYZAAR
  C. ZOSYN
  D. GLUCOVANCE

227. Nonpharmaceutical management to treat constipation should include which of the following?
  A. heating pad
  B. ice packs
  C. increased dietary fibers
  D. massage

228. How would you characterize diverticulitis in regard to its impact on a body part?
    A. stomach
    B. rectum
    C. intestinal tract
    D. ureter

229. Which of the following drugs would you expect as part of the pharmaceutical management for insomnia?
    A. terfenadine
    B. pseudoephedrine
    C. belladonna
    D. zolpidem

230. Which of the following drugs is expected as part of the pharmaceutical management for myocardial infarction?
    A. nizatidine
    B. mipramine
    C. colchicine
    D. warfarin

231. Of the following drugs, which one would be given for glaucoma?
    A. timolol
    B. atropine
    C. tetracaine
    D. prednisolone

232. Which of the following drug types or drug classes is expected to appear in a pharmaceutical management regimen for diabetes mellitus?
    A. ACE inhibitors
    B. hypoglycemic agents
    C. steroids
    D. immunosuppressive agents

233. Gastrointestinal ulcers primarily involve which area of human anatomy?
    A. integumentary system
    B. digestive system
    C. endocrine system
    D. nervous system

✓answers & rationales

1.

B. If the DEA number is missing for a controlled substance, you must call the doctor's office. It is the law that the DEA number appears on a Rx for controlled drugs to avoid drug diversion.

2.

D. The prescription states to give "ibuprofen 400 mg four times a day with food starting now or immediately."

3.

C. For the label, you should never use abbreviations to avoid confusion on the part of the patient and to avoid any liability issues on the pharmacy.

4.

C. The full name allows for assurance that the right patient is getting the right drug. Because there are many people with the same first or last name or even first and last name, the middle name becomes important.

5.

D. The order reads "Discontinue ciprofloxacin, start cephalexin 500 mg by mouth four times a day for 14 days."

6.

A. Script is a short way of saying prescription.

7.

B. The prescription order should provide all the information needed to fill the order properly. Sometimes, you don't have all the info you need and that's when you must call the doctor.

8.

C. The order reads "Give 2 mg of morphine sulfate intravenous push every 2 hours as needed for breakthrough pain for only 9 hours."

9.

D. The term CE means continuing education. These are the credits you need as a technician to get your certification renewed each year. The same goes for the license of a pharmacist. Each state has its own requirements, so you have to check with the State Board of Pharmacy of your state for the correct amount.

10.

C. The codeine part of the drug combo needs to have a "May cause drowsiness" label put on the package. All narcotics can cause drowsiness.

11.

B. The order reads "Alprazolam 0.25 mg by mouth one-time immediately or now."

12.

C. All antibiotic orders need to have a "Finish all medication unless otherwise directed by physician."

13.

C. If you are ever in doubt about an order, you should call the physician's office for verification of the drug and clarification of directions.

14.

A. The order reads "Discontinue hydroxyzine by mouth. Give hydroxyzine 25 mg intramuscularly every 3–4 hours with meperidine intravenously as needed for pain."

15.

A. The best way to give information without the patient forgetting is to put it on the bottle somehow. With an auxillary label, you can do just that, plus the labels are colored and would be able to grab the attention of the patient.

16.

C. The order was missing a frequency. If we know the frequency, then the quantity to dispense can be ascertained by multiplying by 7.

17.

C. The order reads "Famotidine suspension 20 mg by the gastric tube once a day."

18.

D. You would need the amount to be given in order to fill it. The other three items are not necessary to know for filling a prescription. Even if the drug has only one strength, it is still required for the safety of the patient that a specific amount is designated on the script.

19.

C. P.O. means to give it by mouth, so you need to state, "**Take** by mouth."

20.

B. The order reads "Take one tablet by mouth every 4 to 6 hours as needed for headache."

21.

B. For any prescription, you would need the number to dispense, the dosage form, the frequency or specific times of administration, and how it should be given.

22.

A. An external ointment is usually **applied** to the skin.

23.

D. For suppository, you would have to state, "**Insert** into rectum [or anal or vaginal] area."

24.

B. The order states "Take four capsules by mouth now, and in 4 hours, then 100 mg by mouth every 8 hours."

25.

D. A tuberculin syringe contains only 1 cc or 1 ml.

26.

C. For eye drops, the directions should be stated with the word "instill." For example, "Instill two drops in right eye before bed."

27.

B. If you, as a technician, are asked a medical question of any type, you must not answer it and call the pharmacist over to talk to the patient. The pharmacist will make the decision of whether to answer it or refer them to a doctor.

28.

A. The order reads "Take one capsule by mouth every 6 hours as needed for itching."

29.

C. The IV or intravenous route always provides the fastest action since the medication goes directly into the blood stream without having to pass through the liver for metabolism or to circulate through many organs.

30.

B. Albuterol comes as both a tablet and oral inhalation.

31.

D. Ointment jars and dropper bottles are common ways to dispense medication to patients. The different types of dispensing containers depend on the form of the medication.

32.

C. The third ingredient in ROBITUSSIN DAC is pseudoephedrine.

33.

C. P.C. means after meals.

34.

B. PPD is always associated with the drug tuberculin.

35.

D. The label of a bottle contains the drug name, strength, expiration, and other vital info like manufacturer and lot number.

36.

B. If there are missing narcotics, it is important that both the DEA and your State Board of Pharmacy are notified, including some other agencies. However, if there is just a **suspected** diversion, then only the State Board of Pharmacy must be notified.

37.

C. If there is any doubt with a prescription, you should always clarify it before filling it.

38.

A. The direction reads "magnesium sulfate 2 grams intravenously in 100 ml of normal saline to be given over 1 hour."

39.

C. 50% dextrose as a weight-to-volume expression would be 50 gm of dextrose in 100 ml of water. Remember, w/v is gm per 100 ml of volume.

40.

D. Guesswork. Don't ever give a patient something you "guessed" is right.

41.

B. The technician can do everything listed except counsel patients on new medications. Only the pharmacist can do such an act.

42.

D. When reviewing a patient's history, whether in retail or institutional, it is very important to look for allergies or sensitivities to certain drugs and foods. This would have tremendous impact on the compliance for a patient, consequently, successful therapy for the patient.

43.

B. A label dispensed in the hospital setting should contain the patient's name, room number, bed number if needed, and the date it was dispensed.

44.

C. Strip labels is just another source of information regarding proper usage of the drug.

45.

A. The technician's initials are needed when he or she takes part in the filling of the order, whether it be entering it in the computer or counting.

46.

D. MAR stands for medication administration record. It is a very important record in the hospital setting because it has all the medications for a patient, plus time they are to be given and the actual documentation and charting that the nurse did give the drug at a specific time.

47.

D. During any cardiac arrest, the heart stops beating. The first-line drug for that is something to get it "kick started" and that would be epinephrine, a.k.a. adrenaline.

48.

C. Phosphate and calcium will cause a precipitation if mixed together. However, they are frequently added together in a TPN bag. In this case, the calcium should be added first, then the bag shaken or agitated, then the phosphate at the end, and then the bag should be checked for precipitation. At certain concentrations, the two should not be given at all because they would precipitate even if caution is used. The pharmacist should determine this.

49.

C. The directions are "Give meperidine 50 mg intramuscularly every 4 hours as needed for pain."

50.

A. Twice daily after meals is written as "b.i.d. pc."

51.

B. As for eye drops, you need to use the word "instill" in the directions for nose drops.

52.

A. When using an ampule, you should always use a filter needle to withdraw from the ampule or to inject into the bag. You could also use a filter straw, but the straw cannot be injected into a bag, so you must use the straw to withdraw from the ampule.

53.

D. A prescription label should contain the number, patient's full name, directions for use, the doctor's name, date, and name of drug.

54.

D. Age allows the doctor and pharmacist to decide the right dose and which dosage form to use. For example, the dose for a pediatric for TYLENOL is different than for a teenager and a pediatric may need the liquid form due to difficulty in swallowing the tablet.

55.

D. A controlled substance prescription should have the doctor's address, DEA number, and his/her signature.

56.

B. No marks in the refills box leads to assumption of zero refills.

57.

D. There are various ways to tell if a prescription has been tampered. Two of them are listed: quantity is smudged and the ink color is different. However, before accusing the customer of tampering, you should call the doctor's office to clarify any discrepancies.

58.

D. Looking to make sure the patient's name is clear and the drug name and quantity are clear saves time. If the name isn't clear, it's best to ask the patient right then instead of waiting until the prescription is being filled to ask.

59.

D. The DEA number should always be used on a controlled substance order.

60.

D. As stated before, every prescription should have all that is listed in the choices.

61.

C. All the things listed are important for the technician to keep mindful of, but the safety and well-being of the patients are always the top priority of everyone in the health care field.

62.

C. To pick up weights for the torsion balance, you should always use the small tweezer or forcep that comes with the weights, never your fingers and hands.

63.

A. Physicians, osteopaths, dentists, and vets all can prescribe, since they have a degree in medicine or certain types of medicine. However, professional judgment should be used if, for example, you had a dentist prescribe birth control pills. That is outside his scope of practice.

64.

A. Distilled water is commonly used to reconstitute meds that require water, like the suspension forms of AUGMENTIN or AMOXIL. Each of those two require a certain amount of water to be added in order to get it into suspension form before dispensing.

65.

C. Out of the choices listed, the only function relating to product preparation that a tech can perform is retrieving the med.

66.

C. Magnetic carrier transport is not a drug delivery system. Drug delivery systems are methods by which the medication is delivered or transmitted to the patient. The MDI is used for inhalers, the patch is used to have med absorbed from the skin, and the ophthalmic drops are of course a way to get med to the eyes.

67.

C. Grapefruit is the most common of fruits and fruit juices that causes interactions with drugs. Although not many drugs are affected, certain popular drugs

do elicit greater attention for this drug-food interaction.

68.

B. Synergistic drug interaction is when one thing helps increase or enhance the effect of another.

69.

C. To ease withdrawal from a vial, you should always add in the same amount of air equal to the volume you are to take out. In this way, you would maintain the pressure inside the vial so fluid would not squirt back at you.

70.

C. Antagonistic effect is when one drug would cancel or even make worse the effect of another drug.

71.

B. Codeine is a narcotic related to morphine. This would cause drowsiness, regardless of what other drug it is marketed with.

72.

D. When working in a horizontal airflow hood, you should always be working at least 6 inches in from the front edge of the hood in order to maintain sterility.

73.

D. All of the above drug groups listed require monitoring if the patient is also on acetaminophen since they all go through metabolism in the liver.

74.

C. A reason why patients may not comply with directions is that they don't understand them.

75.

B. A hospital pharmacy is considered to be dealing with institutionalized patients.

76.

C. The definition of a solution is that all solutes are dissolved in the solvent.

77.

D. A suspension is when the solute is not entirely dissolved in the solvent and is left suspended in the solution.

78.

C. A community pharmacy deals with ambulatory patients. Ambulatory means walking or walk about.

79.

A. A buffer is used to keep the pH from changing too drastically when acids or bases are added to a mixture.

80.

D. Zileuton (ZYFLO) and Zafirlukast (ACCOLATE) are used to prevent asthma attacks. They do this by inhibiting the effects of leukotrienes on the body.

81.

A. The most important thing to always remember and perform is an aseptic technique. This is the primary way and first step in preventing contamination of the admixture.

82.

A. Syrup contains a lot of sugar and when dealing with diabetics you must be careful with the sugar content.

83.

D. Levigation reduces particle size thereby allowing components to better mix within the suspension.

84.

D. The three sources listed can all contribute equally to the contamination of an IV admixture if the person doing the preparing is not careful.

85.

A. 000 is the largest capsule size. It may seem somewhat contradictory given that 0 is usually designated as being of the lowest value and consequently the smallest.

86.

C. Syrup is the one of the four listed that does not contain alcohol. It contains sugar or an artificial sweetener instead.

87.

C. An aseptic technique, as stated before, is the primary way contamination of IV admixtures is prevented.

88.

C. Levigation is the method by which a large particle is broken down within a cream or liquid substance. It is the attempt of reducing the particle size so the drug could be well mixed and evenly distributed.

89.

A. Glassine paper is the most common type of paper used to weigh drugs. The official definition of the paper is a nearly transparent, resilient, glazed paper resistant to the passage of air and grease.

90.

A. Thinking of this question logically, you would understand that 1L is 1000ml. If you divide 4 into 1000, you would have 250 minutes, which is around 4 hours.

91.

C. For basic pharmacokinetics, the areas that mainly interest the pharmacist and doctors are absorption, distribution, and elimination.

92.

A. The main organs that eliminate drugs are the liver and kidneys. The liver takes care of metabolism and the kidneys the excretion of many drugs.

93.

D. You would have to divide 4000u into 10000u to get 0.4ml.

94.

B. The kidney is the part that handles the elimination of the drug.

95.

C. The liver performs the hepatic biotransformations or metabolism.

96.

B. A traditional TPN would include, but is not limited to, amino acids, dextrose, electrolytes, and vitamins.

97.

A. Insulin is produced from the pancreas, in the islet of Langerhans.

98.

C. Bioavailibility is part of the study of pharmacokinetics, which deals with how much of a drug is available to the body and how fast it reaches the blood circulation.

99.

B. A second name for fats in a TPN is lipids.

100.

D. The maximum amount of time any one TPN bag should be hung is 24 hours in order to avoid introduction of contamination and infection.

101.

A. Passive diffusion occurs when there is a barrier that allows molecules to pass from an area of high concentration to an area of lower concentration.

102.

A. You should expel the excess air from the bag before it is clamped and cut.

103.

B. CLARITIN is a popular drug for allergies. It is available over the counter.

104.

B. HMG-CoA reductase inhibitors are used to treat high cholesterol levels or hyperlipidemia.

105.

C. PROTONIX is the only proton pump inhibitor that is available in IV form.

106.

C. Leukotrienes are associated with asthma.

107.

D. Drugs, depending on the form, have both medicaments and excipients. The medicaments are responsible for eliciting the pharmacologic action.

108.

B. Out of the four listed, VERSED would be the most commonly used drug in surgery.

109.

D. There are many reasons why drugs come in different dosage forms. Three valid reasons are given in choices A–C. Patients of a young age can't swallow well, so there are liquids. Plus, liquids allow the medication to taste better, thereby increasing compliance in children. Since the oral route does reduce the amount of drug available, the IV route allows more drug to be in circulation at a faster rate.

110.

B. An example of a solid dosage form is the capsule.

111.

C. You should always wash your hands each time you leave and go back to the hood. You should never talk or wear jewelry anytime while under the hood. It is recommended that you limit the number of times you leave and reenter the hood in order to limit possible contamination.

112.

D. Each form listed is an example of a topical dosage form.

113.

A. Since high salt content has been implicated in hypertension, it is safe to assume that a patient taking meds for hypertension would have a low-salt diet.

114.

C. The Pharmacy and Therapeutics Committee is the key body in the institutional setting that decides on formulary action.

115.

D. For treatment of *H. pylori,* the three combinations listed all have been proven effective against it. Most ulcers now are caused by *H. pylori,* so having an antibiotic in the drug regimen is beneficial and a must for a cure.

116.

B. The "Take medication as directed" instruction is the most vague of the three. If a doctor does write that, then either the doctor has already told the patient the instructions, in which case the pharmacist would have to make sure the patient knows the instructions, or the drug itself has instructions on how to take it preprinted on the package, like a Medrol DosePak. In either case, the pharmacist must clarify with the patient that he or she understands the correct way to take the drug.

117.

B. A formulary is a list of drugs that a hospital has decided to keep in stock on a regular basis. The formulary is carefully selected in that each drug is analyzed against others to determine the more clinically important ones to carry and which one offers the best cost advantage.

118.

C. A very likely reason for drug errors is the poor legibility of some doctors' handwriting.

119.

B. CARDIZEM's nonimmediate release formulation is designated with the letters CD.

120.

D. The three reasons listed are all areas of consideration to take into account when choosing a drug for the formulary. The process will always go through groups of people and eventually to the P&T committee for approval or rejection.

121.

D. Dispensing errors can occur under many different environments and the three listed are common reasons for them. Even with some of the best, excessive workloads and interruptions can disrupt the thought pattern and cause some unwanted errors. Though dispensing drugs seems simple, the act does take concentration and continual focus on the task.

122.

A. Protein anabolism requires the addition of nitrogen into the diet. Amino acids provide the nitrogen base necessary to create protein.

123.

B. Paste is a topical dosage but it's thicker and has a more solid consistency than ointments or creams.

124.

B. Osteoarthritis is the inflammation of joints but it is also called degenerative joint disease because the joints seem to get weaker and more painful.

125.

D. Hemorrhoids are inflammation in the anal area. Hydrocortisone is present in many suppositories used to treat the condition. Hydrocortisone is a steroid and helps to reduce inflammation.

126.

C. The desired room temperature would be 15–30°C.

127.

A. Since a patient has a pulmonary disease, the obvious choice for a nonpharmaceutical treatment would be to stop smoking.

128.

C. The lungs would be the organs most affected by a restricted pulmonary air flow.

129.

C. Light therapy is assumed to work for depression since it brightens up a room, which is thought to increase mood.

130.

B. Cool compressions should be used to treat a fever because it would bring down the body temperature.

131.

A. Diarrhea can be handled by taking loperamide (IMODIUM). Nizatidine is for ulcers, phenytoin for seizures, and colchicines for gout.

132.

C. Sumatriptan is one of the "triptans" and is used to treat migraine headaches.

133.

A. Constipation can be treated with the use of laxatives.

134.

B. Since ulcers can be caused by food intake, the patient should stay away from irritating foods or foods that can upset the stomach.

135.

D. Phenytoin is used to treat epilepsy. Allopurinol is for gout, lovastatin for high cholesterol levels, and paclitaxel is for ovarian carcinoma.

136.

D. Cyclopentolate is an ophthalmic agent used as a diagnostic agent.

137.

D. Theophylline is a drug used in the management of asthma. Terconazole is an antifungal, terazosin is used to treat benign prostatic hyperplasia or hypertension, and thioridazine is used to manage psychotic disorders.

138.

B. Carboplatin is used to treat various types of cancer. Ciprofloxacin is an antibiotic, celecoxib is for osteoarthritis, and carbamezepine is used for seizures.

139.

C. There is no such thing available that is ferrous hydrochloride.

140.

B. High blood pressure is the common term for hypertension.

141.

C. Cutting back on salt intake would greatly help to control the effects of congestive heart failure since salt has been implicated in many cardiovascular diseases.

142.

B. Diuretics would normally be seen in management of congestive heart failure since excess fluids in the body has been implicated in causing heart diseases.

143.

C. Pamidronate is the drug out of the list of four that is considered a bisphosphonate and used to treat Paget's disease. Pancrealipase is an enzyme supplement, palivizumab is used to treat respiratory syncytial virus in pediatrics, and paclitaxel is a chemotherapeutic agent.

144.

A. Expectorants can be used in helping manage COPD in order to clear any phlegm from the lungs.

145.

A. Depression involves the CNS of the human body.

146.

C. Cirrhosis is associated with a disease of the liver.

147.

C. Antipyretics are agents used to reduce fevers. Anti-inflammatories are used to decrease swelling, antineoplastics are chemo agents, and anticoagulants are used to prevent blood clotting.

148.

D. HALDOL and ZYPREXA are drugs used to treat mental illnesses, like psychotic disorders.

149.

B. Docusate would be seen as a treatment for constipation. Disopyramide is used for treatment of ventricular tachycardia, dopamine is used for cardiovascular and renal conditions, and disulfiram is used for management of alcoholism.

150.

D. The erosion of the lining of the digestive tract affects the esophagus, stomach, and intestine since all three are part of the digestive tract.

151.

C. Divalproex is the only drug listed that has the indication to treat convulsions.

152.

A. Bronchodilators are routinely used to control asthma since they open up the lungs to help increase breathing.

153.

B. Since arthritis is caused by degeneration of joints and leads to joint pain, specific exercise programs targeted at strengthening the joints should be beneficial to the patient.

154.

B. For ondansetron, a regularly scheduled dosing would mean that the patient is getting a chemotherapeutic agent at the same time. Drugs in the same class as ondansetron should not be given on a regular basis just for nausea and vomiting. They are specifically given only for prevention of nausea and vomiting in relation to chemotherapy.

155.

C. Clonidine patches are made to last for 7 days before the need to change it and put on a new one.

156.

C. Ketorolac is an NSAID and is widely known as having the ability to cause ulcers; therefore, you shouldn't give it to a patient with a known history of ulcers.

157.

D. Isosorbide is a drug used to help improve the oxygenation and opens up the blood vessels for better pumping of the blood.

158.

A. Chronic bronchitis, continual inflammation of the bronchioles, is another term used to describe chronic obstructive pulmonary disease.

159.

C. Albuterol is one of the primary drugs used for treatment of COPD because it allows the smooth muscles to relax and leads to opening of the airway.

160.

C. Mestanol and norethindrone are drugs found in combination for use as birth control pills.

161.

B. Since depression is a mental disease, the drugs classified as psychotherapeutic agents would be best to handle the disease.

162.

D. The two primary drugs used to treat fever are acetaminophen and aspirin.

163.

C. Morizine and flecainide are drugs used for treatment of arrythmias.

164.

B. The brain is the organ most directly involved with neurological seizures.

165.

B. Antacids are an old remedy used to treat upset stomachs and are part of drug therapy for ulcers.

166.

A. Epilepsy is characterized by increased levels of neurotransmission, therefore, the CNS is most directly involved with this disease state.

167.

D. The bronchioles are located in the lungs, the organs most affected by their narrowing.

168.

A. Arthritis is characteristically a disease that attacks the joints and causes pain and inflammation.

169.

A. Hemorrhoids could be due to the fact that the bowel movements are too hard and the fecal matter is not soft enough. Increasing fiber in the diet would make the stools softer, leading to less chances of getting hemorrhoids.

170.

D. For hypertension, the three things listed would be a great way to control it without intervention of drugs. Exercising is just one method to control high blood pressure; it also needs to be controlled by watching the diet.

171.

D. Simvastatin (ZOCOR) is an antihyperlipidemic agent used to lower cholesterol.

172.

D. Myocardial infarctions are sometimes called by all three names: MI, heart attack, and infarct.

173.

A. Nitroglycerin allows the blood vessels to widen to allow blood to travel more easily. In an angina pectoris, there is a burning pain in the chest and down the left arm because of difficulty for the heart to pump the blood due to narrow vessels.

174.

D. Trazodone is the only drug of the four that is not used for nausea and vomiting in one capacity or another. Trazodone is DESYREL and is classified as a tricyclic antidepressant.

175.

C. Atherosclerosis is another term for deposits of lipids or cholesterol in the blood vessels and arteries.

Therefore, lovastatin would be one of the possible drugs given for this condition.

176.

C. Sertraline (ZOLOFT) is an SSRI that is very popular for the management of depression.

177.

A. Used topically, tretinoin is for the treatment of acne. So, out of the patient populations listed, teenagers would be the most likely group to use this drug.

178.

B. If a patient has diarrhea, he or she is also losing lots of electrolytes, so a replacement fluid of electrolytes should be given.

179.

C. MAXZIDE is an antihypertensive drug but is a combination drug best put under the heading of a diuretic/potassium-sparing diuretic. The other three drugs all belong to the class of angiotensin II converting enzyme (ACE) inhibitors.

180.

A. Sucralfate is a drug normally used to protect the stomach from ulcers. The drug just coats the stomach and provides a layer of protection.

181.

D. Misoprostol is a drug that is a synthetic prostaglandin used to protect the stomach from ulcers. It can be found in the combination drug ARTHROTEC, which also contains diclofenac.

182.

C. Asthma is a condition where breathing becomes difficult for the patient. The removal of irritants that can cause constriction of the bronchioles would be a good method to control asthma.

183.

C. NSAIDs were one of the first classes of drugs used to treat arthritis since the class of drugs are anti-inflammatory drugs and is a good way to control the disease state.

184.

D. Hemorrhoids involve the veins when they become constricted, causing the skin to develop an inflammation because of poor blood flow.

185.

A. High blood pressure affects mainly the arteries when it becomes harder for the heart to pump the blood.

186.

B. Bisacodyl works by increasing the contractions of the intestine in those with constipation. Methylcellulose and pysllium are bulk laxatives and docusate is a stool softener.

187.

D. Myocardial infarction affects the heart.

188.

B. Beta-blockers are used to control angina pectoris. Beta receptors on the heart have the effect of decreasing heart pumping if activated. By blocking it, the heart would be able to increase the pump action and allow blood to flow faster and better and this would relieve the symptoms of the disease.

189.

D. Nausea and vomiting involve both the CNS and digestive system, the CNS because of certain chemical stimuli and the digestive because of possibly ingesting food that our body does not like, or simply from motion sickness.

190.

A. HMG-CoA inhibitors are drugs used in the management of atherosclerosis because the disease is characterized by high lipid levels and the inhibitors help to decrease the levels.

191.

C. Glucosamine is not a real available form of insulin.

192.

C. Propoxyophene/acetaminophen is DARVOCET and is a pain medication.

193.

D. Tinea pedis is athlete's foot and is caused by a fungus infection. So, you would give the patient an antifungal preparation, preferably one that is topical.

194.

B. Asthma involves mainly the pulmonary system since the lungs are the primary organs affected.

195.

D. Gastroenteritis is a condition where the stomach and the intestine are inflamed and it feels like having a stomach flu.

196.

B. Urinary incontinence is a condition where the patient is unable to control his or her bladder and has to use the restroom very frequently.

197.

C. DETROL is a drug that is used to combat urinary incontinence. ADDERALL is a drug used for attention deficit disorder, TOPROL is used to control hypertension, and ALDOMET is used to also control hypertension but using a different method than TOPROL.

198.

C. Elimination of certain fats and cholesterol from the diet is one way to control high cholesterol levels, as in hypercholesterolemia.

199.

A. The cessation of smoking is one way to treat myocardial infarction because smoking does place added pressure on the heart to pump the blood, leading to heart problems.

200.

C. Restricted coronary blood circulation has the greatest effect on the heart and blood vessels.

201.

A. Antiemetics is the class of drugs used to treat and manage nausea and vomiting.

202.

D. PROGRAF is the drug used to prevent organ rejection in organ transplant cases.

203.

D. Diabetes mellitus involves mainly the endocrine system.

204.

C. BENADRYL is considered a first-generation antihistimine. The difference between it and the other drugs listed, which are considered second generation, is that the second-generation drugs have less or no sedation and drowsiness effect associated with them.

205.

A. The intestines would be affected by constipation or loose stools.

206.

D. Gastroenteritis involves the digestive system, since that is where the stomach and intestines reside.

207.

B. Loperamide (IMODIUM) is the drug out of the four listed that would be used to manage gastroenteritis, since the drug has an effect in the intestinal area.

208.

C. Verapamil is a calcium channel blocker that is used to manage hypertension. Vecuronium is a paralyzing agent used in surgeries, vincristine is an antineoplastic, and valproic acid is used to manage seizures.

209.

C. Lipid disorders can have an effect on the cardiovascular system of the human body since an increase in lipids would force the heart to pump harder and also would cause narrowing of the blood vessels and arteries.

210.

B. KEFLEX is a cephalosporin and the other three antibiotics listed are all part of the fluoroquinolone class.

211.

D. A low-fat diet would be a great way to manage angina pectoris nonpharmaceutically. Low fat would help the heart to beat and pump blood better, therefore causing less chest pain.

212.

C. Prochlorperazine (COMPAZINE) is a common drug used to treat and manage nausea and vomiting. Loperamide is for diarrhea, docusate is for constipation, and prazosin is for management of hypertension.

213.

D. Atherosclerosis is a disease characterized by high levels of lipids and fats in the body. A low-fat diet, weight maintenance, and an exercise program are good ways to keep the levels low and prevent any cardiac problems.

214.

C. Since diabetes is due to too high a level of sugar or glucose, then it would be best to try to restrict the intake of sugars in the diet.

215.

C. Acetaminophen is one of the usual standard treatments for headaches that are not migraines.

216.

B. Out of the four listed, only RONDEC DM does not contain any narcotic of any kind. The other formulations contain either codeine or hydrocodone.

217.

C. Electrolyte replacement is used to manage gastroenteritis because of the diarrhea associated with it, leading to loss of fluid and nutrients.

218.

A. ACCUZYME is a topical debridement agent. The only other topical debridement listed is SANTYL (collagenase).

219.

C. Antianxiety drugs are sometimes given for insomnia. At times, a patient's insomnia is due to high anxiety and nervousness, instead of just simply difficulty falling asleep.

220.

B. Cholesterol is the more common term for lipid, and high cholesterol also means having a lipid disorder.

221.

C. Antihyperlipidemics are given for MI since lowering the level of cholesterol in the body often helps to reduce the risk for MI.

222.

A. Angina pectoris deals with the cardiovascular system of the body.

223.

B. Atherosclerosis is also related to the term "hardening of the arteries" since that is what happens when the cholesterol starts to build up in the arteries.

224.

B. The pancreas has the responsibility in metabolizing carbohydrates.

225.

A. Glyburide (GLYNASE, MICRONASE) is a common drug given for the management of diabetes mellitus. Fluoxetine is used for depression, amlodipine is for high blood pressure, and furosemide is a diuretic used to manage cardiovascular disease.

226.

A. AUGMENTIN also contains the drug amoxicillin, which is combined with clavulanate. HYZAAR has losartan and hydrochlorothiazide and used for hypertension. ZOSYN has piperacillin/tazobactam and is an antibiotic. GLUCOVANCE has metformin and glyburide and is for treating diabetes.

227.

C. Increasing fiber in the diet is a good method in combating constipation.

228.

C. Diverticulitis occurs in the intestinal tract and is an inflammation of diverticulum, especially of the small pockets in the wall of the colon.

229.

D. Zolpidem (AMBIEN) is a very common controlled drug used to manage insomnia in patients.

230.

D. Warfarin (COUMADIN) is a drug used to prevent blood clots and to thin the blood for better blood flow. This would help in MI cases because it would allow blood to be transported without much force from the heart.

231.

A. Timolol (TIMOPTIC) is the one of the four that is usually given for glaucoma. The others also come in ophthalmic form, but are not for glaucoma.

232.

B. Hypoglycemic agents are used to manage diabetes mellitus, since the disease causes a hyperglycemic condition.

233.

B. Gastrointestinal ulcers primarily involve the digestive systems.

5 Medication Distribution and Inventory System

chapter objectives

Students will demonstrate knowledge in the area of:

➤ Purchasing including ordering, vendors, and contracts

➤ Inventory control including ordering levels, expiration dates, and turnover

➤ Preparation and distribution of inventory including drugs, invoice processing, and pricing

DIRECTIONS Each of the questions or incomplete statements below is followed by suggested answers or completions. Select the **one answer** that is best in each case.

1. What is the meaning of the last two digits in the NDC?
   A. identifies the manufacturer
   B. identifies the brand/generic status
   C. identifies the package size of the drug
   D. identifies the list price

2. What is the purpose of a sales invoice?
   A. lists an order for specific merchandise from the supplier
   B. lists slow-moving merchandise to be sold at sale prices
   C. lists the items shipped and the amount due to the supplier
   D. is an inventory sheet used to track merchandise

3. What is a purchase order?
   A. a list of goods available for purchase
   B. an order form used to select items that a retailer wants to buy for resale
   C. an order form requesting the manufacturer's availability for selected merchandise
   D. the bill that accompanies the order

4. Who is the primary source of merchandise for pharmacy retailers?
   A. wholesalers and manufacturers
   B. store-to-store vendors
   C. larger discount stores
   D. warehouse clubs

5. Who pays the freight charges when shipping terms note "FOB shipping point"?
   A. seller
   B. transport company
   C. buyer
   D. post office

6. What special significance do the middle four numbers of the NDC have?
   A. identify the manufacturer
   B. identify the product, form, and strength
   C. identify the product lot number
   D. identify the geographic region for distribution

7. What is meant by the "terms of payment"?
   A. the date by which the buyer must pay for the merchandise
   B. how much the payment will be after deducting discounts
   C. the schedule for payment
   D. the remedies for late payments

8. What does the term "extension" often found on the purchase order mean?
   A. a request for additional time to order merchandise
   B. an extended period to pay for merchandise
   C. Additional pages are needed to order quantities of merchandise.
   D. The quantity ordered times the unit price provides a total cost for the item ordered.

9. A purchase order usually contains the quantity, description, identifying number, and what else for each item ordered?
   A. gross price
   B. total charges
   C. unit price
   D. percent discount

10. Deducting the trade discount from the list price results in what type of price for the retailer?
    A. discount price
    B. net price

C. retail price

D. sales price

11. What is a trade discount?

A. a reduction in the list price

B. savings resulting from a trade between retailers

C. a discount offered based on the type of trade

D. a discount traded for services or merchandise

12. What special importance do the first five digits of the NDC have?

A. identify the manufacturer

B. identify the product

C. identify the lot number

D. identify the year of manufacture

13. What is another term for the suggested retail price?

A. gross price

B. trade price

C. single price

D. list price

14. Who pays the freight charges when shipping terms note "FOB destination"?

A. buyer

B. seller

C. post office

D. transport company

15. What is meant by "FOB" when identified in the shipping terms?

A. free on board

B. forward or backlog

C. freeze original billing

D. none of the above

16. How is the "net profit" determined?

A. income less the deductions of all expenses

B. reconciliation of income less checks written

C. income less gross payroll amounts

D. income less taxes paid

17. The NDC on bulk product labels is an acronym for what?

A. new drug component

B. national drug code

C. new drug commodity

D. national drug compendium

18. Which answer best describes how to purchase C-II drugs?

A. C-II drugs may be ordered from the local wholesaler.

B. Use a Schedule II DEA order form 222, file the order form, and invoice separately from all other purchasing statements.

C. C-II drugs may only be ordered from wholesalers that specialize in these drugs.

D. Order C-II drugs according to the pharmacy's running inventory record for C-II drugs.

19. What does AWP represent when referring to drugs?

A. average wholesale price

B. actual wholesale price

C. average weighted price

D. actual weighted price

20. Who would have the authorization to order C-II drugs?

A. any pharmacy staff member

B. the director of pharmacy

C. the pharmacist in charge

D. both B and C

21. What is a physical inventory?

A. the health status of employees

B. the physical condition of the pharmacy location

C. accountability of the actual items in stock

D. the Board of Pharmacy requirement for compounding equipment

22. What is a periodic inventory?
    A. a monthly accountability of sales activity
    B. accountability for merchandise taken monthly, quarterly, semiannually, or annually
    C. taxes paid semiannually
    D. accountant's reference to a balance sheet

23. What is a perpetual inventory system?
    A. a constant record of items purchased and sold
    B. a record of items for purchase
    C. a record of slow-moving items
    D. sales merchandise

24. What is inventory?
    A. stock that is sale-priced
    B. excess merchandise
    C. merchandise offered for sale
    D. merchandise required to be ordered

25. What is inventory turnover?
    A. the number of times specific items are replaced during a given period
    B. replacement of old items with different items
    C. the number of times a sale must be held to reduce slow-moving stock
    D. the number of new drugs that replace or add to similar types of drugs

26. What system is used to identify all prescription drugs approved by the FDA?
    A. UPS
    B. UPN
    C. NDC
    D. UPC

27. How can most products be identified for inventory?
    A. SKI System
    B. UPC System
    C. UPN System
    D. UPS System

28. Which of the following answers best defines a stock bottle?
    A. a bulk product manufactured in-house
    B. a bulk bottle
    C. fast-moving product
    D. product support by backup stock

29. What is the term that notes the amount a business pays for merchandise, including freight changes and services?
    A. selling price
    B. markup
    C. cost
    D. profit

30. What does the term "markup" mean?
    A. the price charged to the best customers
    B. contract prices
    C. the amount added to the cost of a product
    D. entries to sales records

31. What is the markup formula?
    A. selling price + cost = markup
    B. markup − cost = selling price
    C. cost − markup − discount = selling price
    D. cost + markup = selling price

32. What is meant by retail?
    A. opening a pharmacy
    B. selling goods directly to the customer
    C. reselling goods to institutions
    D. the profit made above wholesale

33. What is wholesale?
    A. engaging in the whole resale of goods to community pharmacies, manufacturers, and the public
    B. the sale of goods at a lower price to retailers who resell the goods to customers at a higher price

C. the selling of goods in "whole" lots only

D. the price the manufacturer charges the public if sold directly

34. What is it called when the expenses exceed the revenues?

A. break-even

B. income

C. loss

D. none of the above

35. What is COGS?

A. counting overstocked goods for sale

B. cleaning of goods on shelves

C. cost of goods sold

D. none of the above

36. What is a markdown?

A. revenue excluded from the purchase price

B. a percentage reduction in price

C. a professional courtesy extended to other pharmacy practitioners

D. a pricing practice used to keep prices stable

37. What are rebates?

A. a return of money for meeting specific conditions

B. a finance charge for late payments

C. specific dates by which payments must be made

D. additional goods supplied as an incentive to purchase larger quantities

38. Which of the following is an important element to look at on the bulk drug label of an incoming order?

A. the condition of the label

B. the name of the drug manufacturer

C. the expiration date of the drug

D. none of the above

39. Why is it important to rotate stock on shelves?

A. prevents dust buildup

B. saves shelf space

C. ensures use of the product with the closest expiration date

D. provides a busy image

40. What is the difference between pricing and reimbursement?

A. Pricing drugs is determined by the retailer, and reimbursement is determined by the third-party payer.

B. Pricing refers to all items and services, while reimbursement refers only to drugs.

C. Pricing and reimbursement are the same.

D. third-party payer's price and retailers receive reimbursement

✓answers & rationales

1.

C. The last two digits always identify the size of the package.

2.

C. Invoices are used to identify what was shipped and the amount the buyer owes the supplier.

3.

B. A purchase order is simply a form or sheet that the buyer uses to record what he or she wants to buy from the supplier.

4.

A. The wholesaler and manufacturer represent the two most predominant suppliers for a pharmacy retailer. The wholesaler buys drugs from various manufacturers and acts as the middleman, while the manufacturer is the direct supplier of drugs and some drugs, like vaccines, sometimes can only be purchased straight from the manufacturer.

5.

C. "FOB" stands for freight on board. If it is FOB buyer, this indicates that once the goods have reached the intended destination, the buyer has to pay for the delivery and shipping charges.

6.

B. The middle four numbers in the NDC identify the product, form, and strength.

7.

A. "Terms of payment" is the date when the buyer must pay for the merchandise. Many times, the payment is set at a certain date in order for the buyer to get a discount on the purchase. If they don't pay by then, then the discount is null and void.

8.

D. The "extension" is simply the total cost of a product. If you wanted to buy 10 vials of a product that costs $7 each, then the extension is $70. It is just the cost multiplied by the quantity purchased.

9.

C. The purchase order would normally also have the unit cost for each item in addition to the ones listed in the question.

10.

B. A deduction of the trade discount from the list price would give you the net price.

11.

A. A trade discount is when the buyer gets a reduction on the price of a product or entire purchase. This is sometimes done if you buy a certain amount in dollars.

12.

A. The first five digits identify the manufacturer.

13.

D. "List price" is another term for the price set by the retailer.

14.

B. The seller pays the freight charges for FOB destination because it designates that once the shipment reaches the destination, then the charges would be paid at that time.

15.

A. FOB stands for free on board. This means that the transportation fee has been or will be paid for and the shipper doing the transport does not incur any charges.

16.

A. Net profit in strict business terms is the total amount of revenue, in most cases income and sales, minus the expense, in most cases cost of inventory and cost of running the business.

17.

B. NDC stands for national drug code. Each bottle or box of medication has a unique NDC number. A box of unit dosed TOPROL XL 50mg tablets has a different NDC from a box of 100 tablets of TOPROL XL 50mg.

18.

B. To order C-II drugs, a DEA form 222 is used and the order form is then filed separately from other drug orders and is usually also received separately from other drugs. The invoices are also kept separately from other drug invoices.

19.

A. AWP is average wholesale price. It usually represents how much a drug would cost a buyer.

20.

D. C-II drug orders are usually initiated by the director of pharmacy or the pharmacist in charge, PIC.

21.

C. A physical inventory is when each single item is counted in the pharmacy and all items in stock are accountable for purposes of financial record-keeping.

22.

B. A periodic inventory is when inventory is taken at certain intervals during the year. Some pharmacies may take inventory annually, semiannually, or even quarterly.

23.

A. A perpetual inventory system is when the drugs are counted on a daily basis and each tablet dispensed or each tablet received is counted each time. Perpetual inventories are constant recordkeeping.

24.

C. Inventory is simply what the retailer has for sale.

25.

A. Inventory turnover is the number of times an item is replaced in a given year or month or a time period that is measured. The higher the number, the more it is bought. Of course, this can sometimes be deceiving because people can steal and this would make it seem like the item is bought.

26.

C. The NDC number represents all drugs approved by the FDA. You would not find NDC numbers on some herbal remedies because the FDA does not approve these drugs.

27.

B. The UPC system represents a way for the products to be identified for inventory. The UPC is a simple bar code that is read electronically.

28.

B. A stock bottle is considered a bulk item because it represents many doses in one container, similar to a MAALOX bottle or CHLORASEPTIC spray.

29.

C. Cost is the total amount that a business pays for an item plus shipment fees.

30.

C. A markup is just the amount of gross profit a business makes when it sells its merchandise or inventory. Businesses add different amounts to the cost of the product to cover overhead and labor costs.

31.

D. The formula for markup is simply: cost + markup = selling price.

32.

B. Retail is the act of selling goods straight to the customer. Retail acts as the middleman between the wholesaler and end buyer or customer.

33.

B. Wholesale is the price that the retailer pays for goods and then the retailer will ultimately charge a markup to the customer at time of sale.

34.

C. If you lose more than you make, then you have a loss. Break-even is when you make as much as it costs you to run the business.

35.

C. COGS is cost of goods sold, which is just how much the retailer pays for the goods.

36.

B. A markdown, opposite of markup, is a reduction in price.

37.

A. A rebate is when the purchaser gets a certain amount of money back if certain conditions and criteria are met.

38.

C. When checking in an order, the expiration date must always be checked to make sure the product is not expired or about to expire. If it is expired or about to be, then it should be returned immediately for a full refund from the wholesaler, if possible.

39.

C. Rotating stock ensures that the product that will expire the earliest is used first.

40.

A. Pricing is an act done by the retailer. Reimbursement is an act done by the third-party insurance company. The price a retailer charges for a drug may not always be paid back in full through a reimbursement from the third-party company. Insurance companies will tend to pay back a little less if it is possible because they would have already done studies and analysis and decided that a drug will get X dollars back. If the retailer charges more than X dollars, then the retailer will probably only get X dollars back regardless of original charge.

6

Management of Facilities, Resources, Information, and Understanding of the Laws Relating to Pharmacy

chapter objectives

Students will demonstrate knowledge in the area of:

➤ management of policies and the retail sector

➤ maintenance of facilities and equipment and records

➤ management of human resources in terms of roles, duties, and responsibilities

➤ electronic and computer information

➤ law relating to statutes, regulations, standards, and ethics as they apply to pharmacy

DIRECTIONS Each of the questions or incomplete statements below is followed by suggested answers or completions. Select the **one answer** that is best in each case.

1. A pharmacy department should be able to provide which of the following management essentials to guide pharmacy activities?
   A. a drug price list
   B. a mission statement
   C. a formulary
   D. a list of pharmaceutical representatives

2. What is the allowable charge?
   A. The allowable charge is the maximum amount that a third-party payer will reimburse a provider or supplier for a service or an item.
   B. The allowable charge is the amount that is charged to the patient.
   C. The allowable charge is the amount applied to a patient's credit card.
   D. The allowable charge is the least amount that a third-party payer will reimburse for an item or service.

3. Basic records for pharmacy include which of the following?
   A. purchase orders
   B. shipping invoices
   C. narcotic forms
   D. all of the above

4. Which of the following is the best description of a salary?
   A. an hourly pay for a specific set of hours worked
   B. variable payments made to employees working split shifts
   C. a contract to keep a payment to an employee set for a specified period of time
   D. a preset amount paid to an employee

5. What should be the foremost purpose of management?
   A. to provide guidance to staff while also motivating them
   B. to implement a Total Quality Environment
   C. to monitor Continuous Quality Improvement
   D. to establish teams and workgroups

6. In the hospital setting, your coworkers would include
   A. just the other members of the pharmacy staff
   B. the pharmacy staff and nursing staff
   C. the staff of pharmacy, nursing, and all those working in the hospital
   D. only those that deliver direct medical care to patients

7. What is an employee's take-home net pay?
   A. the employee's pay reported to the Internal Revenue Service
   B. the pay after income taxes and other deductions are subtracted from gross pay
   C. the portion of an employee's pay set aside for unseen circumstances
   D. new employee tax

8. What does it mean to extend a professional courtesy?
   A. saying "hello" to other health care staff
   B. providing a discount for items purchased by a person in the same field of work
   C. a daily greeting for patients
   D. none of the above

9. What is a payroll?
   A. a list showing names of employees and the amounts paid to each for work performed
   B. the total wages paid out to working staff
   C. a list of full- and part-time employees
   D. a form listing employees submitted to the Internal Revenue Service

10. Who is the person in whose name an insurance policy is held?
    A. dependent
    B. subscriber
    C. beneficiary
    D. patient

11. What method is used to assign budget money for various operations in the pharmacy?
    A. inventory
    B. budgetary balancing
    C. departmental accountability
    D. allocation

12. What does "overhead" include?
    A. lighting
    B. rent, insurance, and utilities
    C. ceilings
    D. the cost for contracts with manufacturers

13. What is the importance of having a budget?
    A. It is required by the Internal Revenue Service.
    B. It plans the pharmacy's future income, costs, expenses, and net income.
    C. It is useful in purchasing merchandise on credit.
    D. It indicates the status of a company's ability to operate.

14. How does the pharmacy receive payment from third-party payers?
    A. The pharmacy submits a purchase order to the third-party payer.

B. The pharmacy submits a Certificate of Medical Necessity to the third-party payer.
    C. The pharmacy submits a claim via the telephone line or other electronic means.
    D. The pharmacy telephones information to the third-party payer.

15. What does a financial statement provide?
    A. the solidness of a company's sales
    B. the assets a company has in savings
    C. status of a company's progress and financial condition
    D. a verification of assets required by the IRS

16. What tools does management use to analyze business performance?
    A. income statements and balance sheets
    B. owner's equity and liability
    C. purchasing invoices
    D. inventory on hand

17. Unless otherwise noted, how should drugs be stored?
    A. in a nonhumid area at room temperature
    B. on shelves
    C. in a medicine cabinet
    D. any place convenient to enable efficient filling and dispensing of drugs

18. The current pharmacy budget is $118,000. What is the new budget resulting from an 11% increase?
    A. $130,780
    B. $130,980
    C. $12,980
    D. $125,000

19. What is the term that expresses the revenue in excess of the cost of the merchandise plus the operating expenses?
    A. markup
    B. profit
    C. net revenue
    D. earnings

20. Some examples of third-party payers include which of the following?
    A. Medicare
    B. Medicaid
    C. insurance companies
    D. all of the above

21. The pharmacy budget for drug purchasing is $85,000. The total pharmacy budget is $112,000. What percent of the budget is devoted to drug purchases?
    A. 24%
    B. 76%
    C. 32%
    D. 85%

22. An important part of a pharmacy operations management includes which of the following?
    A. workflow
    B. monitoring personal leave
    C. compliance with overall facility needs
    D. providing whatever upper management wants

23. Which of the following ways best keeps pharmacy objectives uniform and consistent?
    A. a newsletter
    B. e-mail
    C. journals
    D. a current policy manual

24. What are the two methods of pharmacy claims submission to third-party payers?

A. U.S. Postal Service and FedEx
B. hardcopy and electronic
C. UPS and DHL
D. fax and e-mail

25. How does the pharmacy computer connect to other computers by means of the telephone?
    A. modem
    B. initialization
    C. tutorial programs
    D. CPU

26. What does the gauge of a needle denote?
    A. weight
    B. length
    C. outside diameter
    D. shaft thickness

27. Computers work to do which of the following tasks?
    A. input and output
    B. processing and storage
    C. communications
    D. all of the above

28. What is the benefit of having a facility accredited by an accrediting agency?
    A. An accredited facility has a line of credit.
    B. Accreditation provides official approval to a facility that it meets a set of specific standards.
    C. Accreditation entices more patients to come to the facility.
    D. There is no benefit to being accredited.

29. What is the terminal when referring to computers?
    A. a stand-alone computer
    B. the last entry made to a computer
    C. workstation where data is entered or received
    D. specialized terms used to command computer functions

30. Which sanitizer is commonly used to clean the work surface of the laminar flow hood?
    A. 70% isopropyl alcohol
    B. povidone–iodine solution
    C. 95% ethyl alcohol
    D. hexachlorophene

31. What directs the computer to do specifically designed functions?
    A. the menu
    B. the disk drive
    C. function keys
    D. software

32. What are the special words and symbols called that will perform tasks on the computer?
    A. menu
    B. commands
    C. syntax
    D. graphic utilization integrators

33. What are the parts of a syringe?
    A. reservoir and plunger
    B. cylinder and piston
    C. barrel and plunger
    D. container and head

34. What would be the need for a fast mover or speed shelf?
    A. Reordering drugs is faster.
    B. These shelves are easily removed and placed somewhere else.
    C. Frequently used medications are conveniently accessible.
    D. This area contains only controlled substances for better monitoring.

35. Which of the following is important to have included in a chemo prep kit?
    A. dust/mist respirator
    B. gown

C. gloves
D. all of the above

36. As a group, what is a keyboard, monitor, printer, and CPU called?
    A. input devices
    B. computer hardware
    C. output devices
    D. peripherals

37. What piece of equipment reduces the risk of contamination when preparing IV admixtures?
    A. UV lighting
    B. humidifiers
    C. laminar flow hoods
    D. foot-pedal sinks

38. What is a special secured word to activate a computer called?
    A. tutorial
    B. password
    C. sign on
    D. alpha-numeric byte

39. Why have a tachy mat at the entrance of an IV room?
    A. to post notes for other staff
    B. to reduce particle counts from shoe debris
    C. to leave shoes on while in the IV room
    D. to soften the hard entry to the IV room

40. Which of the following uses is not usual for a spatula?
    A. removing cotton from a stock bottle of medication
    B. mixing ointments
    C. counting tablets and capsules
    D. transferring powders from the stock bottle to the balance

41. In a typical computer setup, which piece of hardware is the output device?
    A. printer
    B. monitor
    C. modem
    D. keyboard

42. What part of the laminar flow hood is responsible for removing microcontaminents?
    A. the prefilter
    B. the plenum
    C. the recovery vent
    D. the HEPA filter

43. Computer technology in pharmacy has had its greatest impact on which of the following?
    A. communications
    B. recordkeeping
    C. distributive pharmacy processing efficiency
    D. all of the above

44. What is essential in order to be prepared for handling cytotoxic drug spills?
    A. latex gloves
    B. disposable, absorbent towels
    C. chemo spill kits
    D. alternate pharmacy workplace

45. What basic areas do typical pharmacy settings have?
    A. a work area, a bathroom, and a coatroom
    B. a work area and a storage area
    C. a storage area and a counseling area
    D. a drug area and a durable medical equipment (DME) area

46. What equipment is available to measure out liquid volumes?
    A. counting trays
    B. graduates
    C. ovals
    D. vials

47. What is a hard copy?
    A. the file on the hard drive
    B. an acetate copy used for overhead projectors
    C. rigid backing for a presentation
    D. information printed on paper

48. On a computer, what are the keys used to perform selective functions?
    A. macro keys
    B. command keys
    C. function keys
    D. icons

49. What type of equipment would you expect to find in a hospital pharmacy work setting but not in the retail pharmacy setting?
    A. computers and printers
    B. laminar flow hood
    C. amber liquid bottles
    D. counting trays

50. What would you likely do to prevent losing information stored on a computer?
    A. Make a backup disk.
    B. File the hard copy of the information.
    C. Save a record file to the hard drive.
    D. Never shut off the computer.

51. What does the term "CPU" stand for?
    A. cleared processing unit
    B. central processing unit
    C. continuous production unit
    D. central production unit

52. What is one of the most important elements in measuring a technician's performance?
    A. size of the pharmacy
    B. competencies in pharmacy tasks

C. work load

D. size of formulary

53. Which of the following is NOT a reason for a rejection of an insurance claim for a prescription?

A. refilled too early

B. incorrect group number

C. drug cost is over $100

D. patient not covered by insurance company

54. Which duties are appropriate to include in a position description for a pharmacy technician?

A. receiving the prescription, interpreting questionable items on the prescription, selecting the drug, labeling the container, and giving the prescription to the patient

B. receiving the prescription, assessing the contents of the prescription, selecting the appropriate drug, labeling the container, and counseling the patient

C. receiving the prescription, reading the contents of the prescription, selecting the appropriate drug, labeling the container, and notifying the pharmacist that the drug is ready to be checked

D. receiving the prescription, reading the contents of the prescription, substituting the drug as needed, labeling the container, and notifying the pharmacist that the drug is ready for approval

55. What are some of the specific criteria that define the pharmacy technician's role?

A. works under the supervision of a pharmacist

B. does not require the use of professional judgment

C. performs duties primarily limited to the distributive pharmacy function

D. all of the above

56. To whom does the term pharmacy "supportive personnel" refer?

A. all personnel who support the pharmacy activity

B. only personnel in the pharmacy department who support the pharmacy activity

C. only pharmacy technicians

D. there is no such reference to personnel

57. A pharmacy technician may perform the following duties except

A. maintaining patient records, filling and dispensing routine orders for stock supplies, and preparing routine compounding

B. prepackaging drugs in single dose or unit-of-use, maintaining inventories of drug supplies, and completing insurance forms

C. providing clinical counseling, providing clinical information to medical staff, and providing patient medical history data to requestors

D. labeling medication doses, preparing intravenous admixtures, and maintaining the cleanliness of laminar flow hood

58. Pharmacy technician duties vary with the type of pharmacy practice. However, the duties common to all pharmacy settings include

A. preparing ophthalmic preparations under the laminar flow hood

B. measuring out the medication, labeling the container, and packaging the medication

C. helping patients find over-the-counter products

D. advising patients about symptoms they are experiencing

59. "Studies in animals or human beings have demonstrated fetal abnormalities or there is evidence of fetal risk based on human experience, or both, and the risk of the use of the drug in pregnant women clearly outweighs any possible benefit. The drug is contraindicated in women who are or may become pregnant" defines which category of fetal risk factors?
    A. X
    B. A
    C. B
    D. C

60. "There is positive evidence of human fetal risk, but the benefits from use in pregnant women may be acceptable despite the risk (e.g., if the drug is needed in a life-threatening situation or for a serious disease for which safer drugs cannot be used or are ineffective)" defines which category of fetal risk factors?
    A. X
    B. B
    C. C
    D. D

61. "Either studies in animals have revealed adverse effects on the fetus (teratogenic or embryocidal, or other) and there are no controlled studies in women, or studies in women and animals are not available. Drugs should be given only if the potential benefit justifies the potential risk to the fetus" defines which category of fetal risk factors?
    A. A
    B. X
    C. C
    D. D

62. "Either animal-reproduction studies have not demonstrated a fetal risk but there are no controlled studies in pregnant women, or animal-reproduction studies have shown an adverse effect (other than a decrease in fertility) that was not confirmed in controlled studies in women in the first trimester (and there is no evidence of a risk in later trimesters)" defines which category of fetal risk factors?
    A. A
    B. B
    C. C
    D. X

63. "Controlled studies in women fail to demonstrate a risk to the fetus in the first trimester (and there is no evidence of a risk in later trimesters) and the possibility of fetal harm appears remote" defines which category of fetal risk factors?
    A. A
    B. B
    C. C
    D. D

64. Which of the first letters of the FDA's basic rating system indicates a drug meets bioequivalence requirements?
    A. A
    B. B
    C. E
    D. none of the above

65. What does the Orange Book code designated as "AA" mean?
    A. no bioequivalence problems in conventional dosage forms
    B. documented bioequivalence problem
    C. meets necessary bioequivalence requirements
    D. testing standards are insufficient for determination

66. What does the Orange Book code designation "BD" mean?

A. no bioequivalence problems in conventional dosage forms

B. documented bioequivalence problem

C. meets necessary bioequivalence requirements

D. potential bioequivalence problem

67. What does the Orange Book code designation "AB" mean?

A. no bioequivalence problems in conventional dosage forms

B. documented bioequivalence problem

C. meets necessary bioequivalence requirements

D. potential bioequivalence problem

68. What does the Orange Book code designation "BP" mean?

A. no bioequivalence problems in conventional dosage forms

B. documented bioequivalence problem

C. meets necessary bioequivalence requirements

D. potential bioequivalence problem

69. What does the Orange Book code designation "BS" mean?

A. no bioequivalence problems in conventional dosage forms

B. documented bioequivalence problem

C. meets necessary bioequivalence requirements

D. testing standards are insufficient for determination

70. What does the Orange Book code designation "B*" mean?

A. no bioequivalence problems in conventional dosage forms

B. documented bioequivalence problem

C. meets necessary bioequivalence requirements

D. requires further FDA investigation and review

71. What does the Orange Book code designation "BX" mean?

A. no bioequivalence problems in conventional dosage forms

B. insufficient data to confirm bioequivalence

C. meets necessary bioequivalence requirements

D. potential bioequivalence problem

72. What does the acronym ASHP represent?

A. American Society of Hospital Pharmacists

B. American Schools of Health Practices

C. Association of Specialty Health Practitioners

D. American Society of Health-Systems Pharmacists

73. Which association best represents the interests of chain drug stores?

A. NABP

B. APHA

C. NCPA

D. NACDS

74. To what does FDA refer?

A. Food and Drug Administration

B. Federal Drug Advocates

C. fosinopril-digoxin-atenolol

D. food drugs and accessories

75. Which of the following information sources provides the best overall drug information?

A. *The Merck Manual*

B. *Dorland's Medical Dictionary*

C. *Drug Facts and Comparisons*

D. answers A and B

76. A Class IV controlled substance is represented by which of the following?
    A. diazepam
    B. propoxyphene
    C. zolpidem
    D. all of the above

77. Which of the following practitioners is typically not authorized to write for legend drugs?
    A. PHARM D
    B. MD
    C. DDS
    D. DO

78. A health care profession's code of ethics should stress which of the following?
    A. a patient's dignity
    B. confidentiality
    C. appropriate payment for services
    D. answers A and B

79. What is a promissory agreement between two or more persons or entities?
    A. contract
    B. consent
    C. precedent
    D. standard of care

80. How many refills are permitted for Class III controlled substances?
    A. 0
    B. 5 renewals within 6 months
    C. 6 renewals within 1 year
    D. 1 per month with prescriber's verification

81. What is the single term for legislative enactments that declare, command, or prohibit something?
    A. suits
    B. subpoenas
    C. torts
    D. statutes

82. Which of the following answers best describes statements made to a person in a position of trust, such as an attorney or health care practitioner?
    A. confidentiality
    B. privacy
    C. privileged communication
    D. reasonable care

83. What definition best describes malpractice?
    A. the legal concept of cause and effect
    B. professional negligence, improper discharge of professional duties, or a failure of a professional to meet the profession's standard of care, which results in harm to another
    C. acts performed or omitted that a reasonably prudent health care practitioner would have done or not done under the same or similar situation
    D. the legal rights and duties of private persons

84. In which controlled substances schedule will you find meperidine?
    A. Schedule II
    B. Schedule III
    C. Schedule IV
    D. Schedule V

85. What is a suit?
    A. a court order that requires a person to appear in court to give testimony
    B. a court proceeding that seeks damages and other legal remedies
    C. a legal or civil wrongdoing committed by a health care practitioner
    D. a previous decision that serves as the authority for a similar case

86. What is a subpoena?
    A. a court order that requires a person to appear in court to give testimony
    B. a court proceeding that seeks damages and other legal remedies
    C. a legal or civil wrongdoing committed by a health care practitioner
    D. a previous decision that serves as the authority for a similar case

87. What does confidentiality mean to the pharmacy technician?
    A. maintaining the privacy of a patient's medical history
    B. keeping a pharmacy technician's salary private
    C. the pharmacy supervisor having confidence in the pharmacy technician
    D. being able to complete third-party payer forms in any environment

88. What is the function of the State Board of Pharmacy?
    A. to regulate pharmacy practice
    B. to inspect pharmacies for compliance with pharmacy laws and regulations
    C. to revoke or suspend the pharmacy license of practitioners found guilty of violating pharmacy laws or regulations
    D. all of the above

89. In which controlled substances schedule will you find ketamine?
    A. Schedule V
    B. Schedule IV
    C. Schedule III
    D. Schedule II

90. NORCO is a controlled drug because it contains this ingredient.
    A. codeine
    B. hydrocodone
    C. morphine
    D. carisoprodol

91. On a drug bottle, what would designate that the drug is a legend drug as opposed to an OTC drug?
    A. "Warning: May be habit forming."
    B. "RX Only"
    C. "Note: Original date of manufacture is MO/DAY/YR."
    D. "Caution: Federal law prohibits dispensing without a prescription."

92. When can the generic form of a drug be produced?
    A. anytime
    B. when the brand-name patent expires
    C. FDA determines production for generics
    D. generic drug manufacturers determine when to produce generic drugs

93. In which Schedule of controlled substances will you find oxycodone?
    A. Schedule I
    B. Schedule II
    C. Schedule III
    D. Schedule IV

94. Which answer best describes how often a C-III and C-IV drug may be refilled?
    A. PRN
    B. All refills must be called in to the prescriber and verified.
    C. one refill every 30 days for up to 1 year
    D. Five refills within 6 months may be authorized by the prescriber.

95. Which answer best describes the information that should be included in a Schedule V sales log for C-V drugs sold without a prescription?
    A. dispensing date, printed name, signature and address of buyer, name and quantity of the product sold, and the pharmacist's signature
    B. dispensing date, signature and phone number of buyer, the product name, and the product company with lot number
    C. dispensing date, signature of buyer, name and quantity of product sold, price of the product sold, and the lot number of the product sold
    D. dispensing date, buyer signature, pharmacist signature, product name and amount, and the expiration date of the product

96. DURAGESIC patch would be in which schedule?
    A. I
    B. II
    C. III
    D. not a controlled drug

97. What does Schedule I tell us about a drug?
    A. The drug has a high potential for abuse and physical or psychological dependence.
    B. The drug has a moderate or low potential for physical dependence and a high potential for psychological abuse.
    C. The drug has limited potential for physical or psychological dependence.
    D. The drug has no currently accepted medical use in the United States because of its high potential for abuse.

98. How many refills are permitted for a Schedule II controlled substance?
    A. 0

B. 1
C. 2
D. 3

99. Which answer best describes when a Schedule II prescription may be honored as a verbal order?
    A. never
    B. in an emergency
    C. There are no stipulations as long as you can acknowledge the prescriber by his/her DEA number.
    D. in an emergency as long as only the required quantity is dispensed and the prescriber follows up with a written and signed prescription within a specified time frame

100. Is a pharmacy allowed to partially fill a C-II prescription?
    A. yes, but each state has its own regulations for this act
    B. no for every state
    C. yes, but only limited to certain C-II drugs
    D. yes, but only allowed to be done on certain days of the week

101. What does C-III tell us about a drug?
    A. The drug has a high potential for abuse and physical or psychological dependence.
    B. The drug has a moderate or low potential for physical dependence and a high potential for psychological abuse.
    C. The drug has limited potential for physical or psychological dependence.
    D. The drug has a limited potential for abuse.

102. What does C-II tell us about a drug?
    A. The drug has a high potential for abuse and physical or psychological dependence.

B. The drug has a moderate or low potential for physical dependence and a high potential for psychological abuse.

C. The drug has limited potential for physical or psychological dependence.

D. The drug has a limited potential for abuse.

103. The original date for a VALIUM script was 6/1/02. The patient is allowed two refills on it. He comes for the second refill on 1/10/03. Should the pharmacist refill it?

A. Yes, one refill is left

B. No, VALIUM should only be allowed one refill

C. No, it is past 6 months

D. Yes, because the scrip automatically renews the next year

104. What does C-IV tell us about a drug?

A. The drug has a high potential for abuse and physical or psychological dependence.

B. The drug has a moderate or low potential for physical dependence and a high potential for psychological abuse.

C. The drug has limited potential for physical or psychological dependence.

D. The drug has a limited potential for abuse.

105. What does C-V tell us about a drug?

A. The drug has a high potential for abuse and physical or psychological dependence.

B. The drug has a moderate or low potential for physical dependence and a high potential for psychological abuse.

C. The drug has limited potential for physical or psychological dependence.

D. The drug has a limited potential for abuse.

106. How is DARVON different from DARVOCET-N-100?

A. DARVON contains more propoxyphene than DARVOCET.

B. DARVON has acetaminophen and DARVOCET does not.

C. DARVOCET contains acetaminophen and has more propoxyphene than DARVON.

D. DARVOCET is controlled and DARVON is not.

107. Which agency regulates controlled substances?

A. Food and Drug Administration

B. Public Health Service

C. Drug Enforcement Agency

D. Bureau of Narcotics and Dangerous Substances

108. Which drug listed is not a controlled substance under federal law, but many institutions and states do handle it as a controlled drug?

A. AMBIEN

B. PROVIGIL

C. STADOL

D. NUBAIN

109. ERYTHROCIN is to a brand name as erythromycin is to what?

A. proprietary name

B. patent name

C. generic name

D. trademark name

110. Which of the following products is/are exempted from being dispensed in child-resistant containers?

A. diltiazem

B. nitroglycerin sublingual tablets

C. atenolol

D. answers A and C

111. What should you do if you provide a non-controlled substance copy of a prescription to another pharmacy?
    A. It depends on the state's pharmacy regulations.
    B. Cancel the original prescription.
    C. Write up a new prescription.
    D. Enter the date and pharmacy you are providing the prescription and your initials.

112. Which of the following is an example of a Schedule II controlled substance?
    A. chloral hydrate
    B. paregoric
    C. fentanyl
    D. diazepam

113. Which of verbal, faxed, and in-person prescriptions can be handled by the pharmacy technician?
    A. verbal
    B. faxed
    C. in-person
    D. It depends on each state's pharmacy practice guidelines.

114. You receive a script for RITALIN tablets with two refills. What should the pharmacist do?
    A. fill it provided that the script is entirely valid
    B. reduce the refills to only one
    C. not fill it because it is invalid with two refills written
    D. fill it but give the amount plus two refills at one time

115. How are stock bottles of controlled substances distinguishable?
    A. The bottle contains a tamper-proof seal.
    B. Controlled substances may be purchased from specialty wholesalers who provide controlled substances information on the invoice.
    C. The label indicates a "C" and Roman numeral classification from II through V.
    D. The stock bottles may only be prepared in quantities of 90 to allow for a smaller-sized bottle.

116. Which of the following is an example of a Schedule III controlled substance?
    A. acetaminophen with codeine
    B. oxycodone with acetaminophen
    C. oxazepam
    D. guaifenesin with codeine

117. In addition to the information typically found on a prescription order, the following information is required for all prescriptions for controlled substances:
    A. patient's age, patient's gender
    B. patient's address, prescriber's DEA number
    C. patient's address, responsible payer
    D. prescriber's specialty, diagnosis

118. What should you consider when dealing with an elderly patient?
    A. hearing ability
    B. chronic conditions
    C. multiple drug management
    D. all of the above

119. What is verbal communication?
    A. messages transmitted through body motions
    B. messages delivered through touch
    C. messages transmitted the same as non-verbal communication
    D. messages using words

120. Which of the following best describes the attributes of an effective communicator?
    A. listens to the patient's concerns

B. observes the patient for clues

C. explains information on a level understood by the patient

D. all of the above

121. What is effective communication?

A. messages sent appropriately

B. messages interpreted by the sender

C. messages sent, received, and understood as the sender intended

D. ongoing transmission of messages

122. Which of the following are references to common descriptions of two general types of patients who need pharmacy services?

A. the elderly and women

B. pediatrics and women of child-bearing age

C. travelers and vacationers

D. ambulatory and institutionalized

123. Which of the following best describes communications?

A. directions provided on a prescription label

B. an exchange of messages through verbal and nonverbal methods

C. counseling offered by the pharmacist

D. questions asked by the patient or caregiver

124. What is the importance of providing the patient with complete and understandable information about the directions and use of medications?

A. It avoids potential misuse.

B. It is required by State Boards of Pharmacy.

C. It helps achieve the best therapeutic outcome.

D. answers A and C

125. Which of the following would be included in nonverbal communications?

A. body movements

B. facial expressions

C. hand motions

D. all of the above

126. Which of the following best describes proper telephone answering?

A. Identify yourself and your organization.

B. Get to the point immediately.

C. Request the caller's phone number.

D. Answer "hello" and permit the caller to proceed.

127. What is appropriate telephone etiquette when you put a person on "hold"?

A. Tell the person he or she must hold.

B. Switch to online music.

C. Assure the person that you will return.

D. Let the person know you are busy.

128. Which of the following is not a violation of a patient's right to confidentiality and privacy?

A. leaving the patient's chart open to the public

B. talking about a patient on the elevator

C. telling anyone who asks about the patient the diagnosis or treatment of care

D. withholding information from anyone who calls about the patient

129. Which of the following acronyms represent professional pharmacy associations?

A. NAMES, ASPEN

B. AMA, AHA

C. APhA, NCPA

D. HCFA, HIDA

✓answers & rationales

1.

B. A mission statement allows the employees of the pharmacy to understand the direction and goals of the pharmacy. The statement should include more than just basic rhetoric of pharmacy practice. It should state clearly how and what will be done to promote patient care and to be successful. The statement, above all else, reflects what management truly believes and what is at the core of the business from all strategic points of view.

2.

A. The allowable charge is simply the max that the third party will pay the retailer, in this case the pharmacy. Most insurance companies already set a price for most drugs and no matter how much a pharmacy charges for a drug, there is a specific ceiling that the insurer will not go past.

3.

D. Pharmacy is, to the annoyance of many, a professional that requires a great amount of recordkeeping. All records, including purchase orders, narcotic forms, and shipping invoices, must be kept and accounted for if they have anything dealing with drugs, especially controlled drugs.

4.

D. A salary is an amount of money set forth by the employer and accepted by the employee in return for services rendered.

5.

A. The primary purpose of management is always to provide stable leadership and to encourage the staff to exceed all expectations while developing a good working environment.

6.

C. Coworkers in the institutional setting include all those employees that work there. The nurses, janitors, doctors, clerks, and everyone who is employed there are all your coworkers. This must be remembered because in order to deliver good patient care, it takes all those, whether they have direct or indirect patient contact, to be working together and to support one another. This is more often forgotten than remembered in the work setting.

7.

B. Net pay is what is left after taxes are subtracted from the original salary and wage. In order to minimize taxes paid, it is best to put as much into a pre-tax 401K as a person wishes. This would minimize taxes and help to save for future retirement.

8.

B. Professional courtesy is when you are offered a reduction on costs or you offer a reduction because of jobs in the similar field or occupation.

9.

A. Payroll is simply a list of your human capital expenses. It lists all those employees who work at a specific place and department and also lists their compensation amount.

10.

B. The subscriber is the name of the person who holds the insurance policy. The beneficiary is the person who would get a set amount of money in the event of the death of the subscriber.

11.

D. Allocation is a process whereby a total amount of money of an institution is dispersed among the different departments.

12.

B. Overhead includes rent, insurance, utilities, and all the requirements needed to operate a business physically.

13.

B. A budget helps to allocate expenses and costs in a fair and controllable method and is aimed at reducing indiscriminate spending.

14.

C. In today's society, a pharmacy receives payment by submitting a claim via the telephone line as the prescription is being filled.

15.

C. A financial statement provides an indication of the financial health of the pharmacy and how it is doing now or last year.

16.

A. Balance sheets and income statements are the primary method that any company uses to diagnose the health of a company and the first step in figuring out what to fix if there are any problems financially.

17.

A. Drugs should usually be stored in a nonhumid area at room temperature unless stated otherwise by the manufacturer.

18.

B. This is a basic algebraic problem similar to ones in the calculation section of the book. You can set up the problem as this: 11% = 0.11. Since they are asking for an increase, you would multiply (0.11) ($118,000) = $12,980 + $118,000 = $130,980.

19.

B. The amount of revenue you are able to obtain after taking away the cost of inventory and operating expenses is simply the profit of the company or store.

20.

D. The three choices listed are all examples of third-party payers. By definition, third-party payers are those involved with helping out the customer in obtaining their medications by subsidizing some of the cost.

21.

B. This is simply a division problem: $85,000/ $112,000 = 0.76, or 76%.

22.

A. The workflow of the pharmacy business is a very vital aspect of management because it determines how the pharmacy will be run from day to day and the efficiency of your staff in doing their job.

23.

D. The policies and procedures of not just the pharmacy but also of the hospital as a whole should be kept up to date and be communicated continuously with the staff under the objectives and the purposes of their job.

24.

B. The submission of third-party claims is either done electronically or by mailing off a hard copy to the insurance company.

25.

A. This is not a pharmacy question; it's a tech question. For all of us who have used the Internet, the computer connects to the telephone line via a modem.

26.

C. For needles, the gauge designates how wide the outside diameter is.

27.

D. Computers are made to execute all of the choices listed. They are needed for input and output. The processing speed of it helps to efficiently run a pharmacy while the amount of information it can store helps to keep patient info updated. Plus, computers have become a primary mode of communication over the last decade.

28.

B. The accreditation allows the public and those who work there to know that the hospital meets a certain level of standard of care and to affirm that the facility has the ability to adequately treat those patients who enter the building.

29.

C. A terminal is the workstation where data is entered or received. It is where the majority of the orders are entered in a pharmacy.

30.

A. The sanitizer commonly used to clean the hood is 70% isopropyl alcohol. Sterile water does not provide the decontamination that 70% iso alcohol provides. The others listed are good antiseptics but not good enough for aseptic technique.

31.

D. Software is what tells the computer to do specific functions and to perform certain manipulations.

32.

B. The commands are what is inputted in order to tell the computer to perform certain tasks.

33.

C. The barrel and plunger are names of the parts of a syringe.

34.

C. The fast mover or speed shelf is established within pharmacies to allow easy accessibility and to allow work to flow much more efficiently.

35.

D. The chemo spill kit should contain all of those items listed, dust respirator, gown, gloves, adsorbent mats, signs to identify the area as contaminated, and chemo bags.

36.

B. The keyboard, monitor, printer, and CPU are all considered the hardware of the computer system.

37.

C. Laminar flow hoods greatly decrease risk of contamination through the control of air flow in and out of the room.

38.

B. The password is what is used to control the security of computer access for each individual user.

39.

B. A tachy mat is used to hold particles to it as a person enters a room. This would reduce the possibility of contamination when performing IV admixing.

40.

A. A spatula is not often used to remove cotton from bulk bottles. Tweezers or a rod with a curved or pointed end should remove the cotton.

41.

A. The printer is what is used to produce the output needed. You would input data through the keyboard and output data through the printer.

42.

D. The HEPA filter is the component of the flow hood that is used to remove microcontaminents. The filter allows the air to flow free of particles that could contaminate the sterile environment.

43.

D. Computer technology has impacted various aspects of pharmacy practice. It has improved communication, such as to third-party providers for coverage information, helped recordkeeping to be more efficient and less cumbersome, and has improved overall pharmacy efficiency.

44.

C. A spill kit is the first-line agent used to handle chemo spills. It is very important and is required by law to be available in areas that utilize antineoplastic agents.

45.

B. Taking all the different pharmacy settings into account, the two areas that are common to all is a work area and a storage area. There are areas that appear in the retail setting but not in the institutional setting, like a counseling area.

46.

B. Graduates are used to measure liquid volumes. They are either straight cylindrical shaped or are curved.

47.

D. Hard copy is information printed on paper. For any important information or forms, there should always be a hard copy available and filed away somewhere just in case there are problems with the computer system.

48.

C. The function keys are used to perform functions that are not available on the standard set of keys. Each software application would have a different function for each function key.

49.

B. A laminar flow hood would not be found in the retail setting, only in the hospital or institution setting.

50.

A. In order to prevent a loss of information, you should always make a backup disk of the activities performed for a specific period of time.

51.

B. The CPU is the central processing unit. It is the brains and power source of a computer system.

52.

B. There are various ways to measure the performance of an individual. For the pharmacy setting, it is quite obvious that the competencies of the pharmacy tasks would be the primary way a technician's performance is measured.

53.

C. The cost of a prescription is not a reason why an insurance company rejects a prescription. However, the price of prescription may not be paid in its entirety by the third party. If the company believes that a generic could have been used, it may only pay for the generic cost if a brand was dispensed.

54.

C. This choice is the only choice that does not have activities that should only be performed by the pharmacist. As can be seen, the duties of a technician are many and should be only those duties where personal judgment or the use of clinical information is not required.

55.

D. The choices listed are all criteria that define what a tech can and cannot do.

56.

A. Supportive personnel refer to all those who have direct responsibility in the proper functioning of the pharmacy. This would include pharmacists, technicians, and clerks or stockers.

57.

C. As can be seen by the various duties listed in the choices, this choice is the only one that lists those duties that require clinical judgment calls and the use of medical information to perform the duties.

58.

B. Common pharmacy duties to all settings include measuring out the appropriate amount of medication, container labeling, and placing the medication in the appropriate package.

59.

A. The rating described is that of X. It is the worst rating a drug can receive with respect to effects on pregnancy and the fetus. The most famous drug to have this rating and yet still is in use for leprosy is thalidomide.

60.

D. The rating of D is also a very bad rating, but the risk versus benefit factors should be weighed in order to make the appropriate decision. Is the risk on the fetus justified by the benefit of the drug to the woman?

61.

C. This is the mid range of severity. The C rating is given if no human testing was done, but animal testing has shown adverse effects on the fetus. Once again, the risk versus benefit should be analyzed.

62.

B. The B rating is where the drug is considered safe for use on humans because the animal studies have not revealed any harm to the fetus, but no tests on humans have been done.

63.

A. This is the best rating a drug can get. It states that tests on human subjects have not caused harm to the fetus in the early stage of pregnancy.

64.

A. The FDA's rating system has the A as indicating that a generic drug has been shown to meet bioequivalency requirements as compared to the brand.

65.

A. AA is the best rating a generic drug can get. It means that there are no problems with bioequivalence in the standard dosage forms.

66.

B. BD means that the bioequivalence of the generic does not meet with the brand.

67.

C. AB is a step below AA but still means that bioequivalency is maintained and the generic is comparable to the brand.

68.

D. BP designates that there is potential bioequivalence problems. This means the drug could be equivalent to the brand, but more than likely it is not.

69.

D. BS designates that the drug has been through testing but the data is insufficient to determine if it is perfectly bioequivalent to the brand.

70.

D. B* means that the drug will need more FDA study and review before a final designation is made.

71.

B. BX means that there is simply not enough data to determine equivalency or not.

72.

D. ASHP is a national group of pharmacists that stands for American Society of Health-System Pharmacists. It is one of the largest pharmacist associations in the country.

73.

D. NACDS stands for National Association of Chain Drug Stores and it represents those pharmacists who work in drug stores.

74.

A. FDA is the federal governing body concerned with drugs and medical equipment. It stands for Federal Drug Association.

75.

C. *Drug Facts and Comparisons* is probably the most widely used and trusted of all reference books to be found in a pharmacy. It is very detailed and easy to use as compared to other books.

76.

D. Diazepam, propoxyphene, and zolpidem are all Class IV drugs.

77.

A. Pharm D stands for Doctor of Pharmacy but the degree does not typically allow the person to prescribe drugs, as an MD is allowed to.

78.

D. As health care providers, it is the responsibility of everyone to protect the confidentiality and, in the process, to protect the dignity of the patient.

79.

A. A contract is a legal promise or agreement that binds two or more parties together for a certain action or event.

80.

B. Class III drugs are allowed to have five refills within a 6-month period. If the 6-month period expires before all five refills are taken, then the patient loses the refills that are left.

81.

D. Statutes are legislative enactments that have the force of law and compel the public to be prohibited from doing something or command them to do something.

82.

C. Privileged communication is when a patient allows a certain person to know facts that are very personal and yet important to the administration of care to the patient.

83.

B. Malpractice is a term applied to professionals who improperly performed their duties or have given care that is insufficient or not up to the standards set forth in general practice. It covers lots of different areas. The patient has to have been harmed or the omission of a certain common act has continued to lead to the patient's suffering.

84.

A. Meperidine, or DEMEROL, is a class II narcotic that is similar to morphine.

85.

B. A suit is when a patient or patient's representative takes a caregiver to court to prove damages and neglect and to get a remedy, mostly monetary in nature, from the caregiver.

86.

A. A subpoena is a legal court order requiring a person to appear in court.

87.

A. Confidentiality means to a technician, as to all other health professionals, that there must be a certain level of confidentiality and privacy maintained with regard to a patient's medical information.

88.

D. The State Board of Pharmacy is a government entity with the responsibility of regulating pharmacy practice, inspection of pharmacies for compliance with state and federal laws, to police and act as a watchdog over pharmacists and take action as needed in terms of violations, and many other duties.

89.

C. Ketamine is listed as a Schedule III drug.

90.

B. NORCO contains the ingredient hydrocodone, which makes it a controlled substance.

91.

B. A prescription-only drug would have the label "RX Only" printed on the bottles. Choice D used to be the designation, but was just recently changed to "RX Only."

92.

B. A generic form of a drug can only be produced after the brand name patent expires.

93.

B. Oxycodone, found in PERCOCET or PERCODAN, is a class II drug.

94.

D. For C-III–C-IV, the law states that the patient is allowed five refills within a 6-month period before the prescription is invalid. If 6 months pass and the patient hasn't taken all the refills, then the patient forfeits the remaining refills.

95.

A. If a C-V drug is sold without a prescription, the date it was dispensed, name and signature of the patient, address of the purchaser, the name and amount of the product, and the pharmacist who sold it must be logged in a book.

96.

B. DURAGESIC patches contain the drug fentanyl, a C-II.

97.

D. C-I drugs are those that are considered elicit because they are not considered having medicinal use and have a high potential for abuse.

98.

A. C-II substances are permitted 0 refills.

99.

D. Verbal orders for C-II are only acceptable in an emergency situation. The amount to be dispensed is limited to the amount for the immediate emergency period. The doctor must follow up with a written order within a specified time frame as required by the state the doctor practices in.

100.

A. C-II scripts are allowed to be partially filled, but the amount of partial fill is regulated by each state's pharmacy laws.

101.

B. C-III means that a drug has a moderate or low potential for physical dependence and a high potential for psychological abuse.

102.

A. C-II means that the drug has a high potential for abuse and physical or psychological dependence.

103.

C. VALIUM is a C-IV drug that is allowed five refills in a 6-month period. Although one refill remains, the 6-month period is expired, so the pharmacist should not fill it again.

104.

C. C-IV tells you that there is a limited potential for physical or psychological dependence.

105.

D. C-V is considered to have limited potential for abuse.

106.

C. The difference between DARVOCET and DARVON is two-fold. DARVOCET N 100 has more propoxyphene than DARVON and DARVOCET has acetaminophen, while DARVON is just simply propoxyphene alone.

107.

C. The Drug Enforcement Administration, or DEA, regulates controlled substances.

108.

D. NUBAIN is not a federally controlled substance, but many states and institutions do handle it as a controlled substance.

109.

C. Erythromycin is the generic name to the ERYTHROCIN brand name.

110.

B. Nitroglycerin sublingual tablets are exempted from a child-resistant cap because they are used for chest pains. If a patient has chest pains, it would be hard for them to open the resistant cap.

111.

A. For this situation, the individual laws that govern the practice of pharmacy for each state would apply.

112.

C. Fentanyl is a popular C-II drug used in surgeries and other invasive procedures.

113.

D. Once again, the individual state laws should be consulted with regard to what a technician can and cannot do with a prescription.

114.

C. The pharmacist should not fill it and should contact the doctor about the two refills and file it away in the pharmacy. The patient should be notified of the error and told to see the doctor in order to obtain a new, valid script.

115.

C. The stock bottles of controlled substances are noticeable by having a C printed on them with the Roman numerals II–V on it.

116.

A. Acetaminophen with codeine is an example of a C-III. This could be TYLENOL #3 or #4, depending on the amounts of each drug.

117.

B. The patient's address and prescriber's DEA number must appear on controlled substances.

118.

D. Elderly patients tend to have hearing difficulty, chronic conditions, and/or a long list of drugs that they have to take. Each of these conditions play a large part on their therapy and well-being and must be taken into consideration when dealing with them.

119.

D. Verbal communication is the interaction with others using simply spoken words.

120.

D. An effective communicator is one that not only is able to explain a situation that the patient would understand but is also able to listen and find the clues to what the patient is saying or is not saying. Many patients will be asking for information or expressing their concerns. It is important that they are treated with concern and understanding.

121.

C. In order to communicate something effectively, the message has to have been sent and received as the sender intended the message to be sent.

122.

D. The two general types of patients that a pharmacy would see are those who are ambulatory, walk-ins like in the retail setting and the institutionalized types, or those who are in hospitals.

123.

B. Communication is simply the exchange of thoughts and ideas through a verbal or nonverbal medium.

124.

D. Providing the patient with the most complete information would avoid misuse and achieve the best outcome possible for that patient.

125.

D. Nonverbal communication includes all of the four items listed. It is an act that does not include the act of speaking.

126.

A. When answering the phone, it is important that you identify who you are and where or what department you are working in.

127.

C. When you place a person on hold, you must always state that you will be gone or it will take a certain amount of time and you will return to them at that time.

128.

D. There are many instances where the patient's information and privacy can be compromised. It is important that we as health care providers practice proper ethics and protect that privacy of the patient. The act of withholding information from those who call, even family members, is one way to protect the patient. It would be best to tell those that call that they should talk with the patient directly or to see the patient's doctor in order to get the information they need.

129.

C. APhA stands for American Pharmaceutical Association, while NCPA stands for National Community Pharmacists Association.

Index

A

Abbreviations, medical/pharmaceutical, 124–147
ABELCET, 13, 61
ACE inhibitors, 16, 18, 28, 35, 63, 65, 72, 77
Acetaminophen, 32, 33, 75, 156, 176
Acetazolamide, 23, 69
Acronyms, 124–147
ACTOS, 41, 81
ACULAR, 49, 86
ADALAT, 3, 54
Albuterol, 152, 164, 174, 182
ALDACTONE, 14, 62
ALEVE, 132, 144
ALLEGRA-D, 15, 63
Allopurinol, 31, 36, 50, 74, 78, 87
Alprazolam, 25, 70
ALTACE, 34, 76
Ambulatory care, 127, 140
American Society of Health-System
    Pharmacists, 203, 215
Amikacin, 42, 82
Aminoglutethimide, 28, 72
Amiodarone, 8, 9, 17, 58, 64
Amlodipine, 40, 80
Amoxicillin, 6, 17, 32, 39, 43, 51, 56, 65, 75, 80, 82, 88
Amphoterecin B, 22, 68
ANAPROX, 6, 56

Angina pectoris, 166, 182
Angioplasty, 129, 141
Angiotensin converting enzyme, 130, 143
Angiotensin II receptor antagonists, 125, 139
Antagonistic effect, 156, 176
Anticoagulant, 19, 66
Antipyretics, 163, 181
Antispasmodic, 13, 62
ARICEPT, 14, 62
Arrythmias, 165, 182
ARTHROTEC, 26, 71
ASO (automatic stop order), 126, 140
Aspirin, 47, 49, 85, 86
Asthma, 159, 162, 164, 166, 178, 181, 183
Atherosclerosis, 166, 182
AVAPRO, 10, 59
AXID, 35, 77
Azathioprine, 21, 67
Azelastine, 45, 49, 84, 86
Azithromycin, 40, 80
Azoles, 16, 64

B

Bacteremia, 127, 140
BACTRIM, 8, 57
Barbiturates, 8, 57
Benzodiazepines, 5, 56
Benzonatate, 37, 79

Beta-blockers, 41, 81
BETADINE, 30, 74
Betamethasone, 19, 66
BIAXIN, 10, 59
Blood cells, 129, 142
Bradycardia, 132, 144
Brand medications, 1–52
BRICANYL, 44, 83
Bronchodilator, 35, 77
Bupropion, 12, 61

C

Calcium acetate, 16, 51, 64, 88
Calcium channel blockers, 29, 73
CAPOTEN, 11, 59
Captopril, 16, 22, 41, 46, 47, 64, 68, 81, 85
CARAFATE, 2, 53
Carboplatin, 162, 180
CARDIZEM, 161, 179
CARDURA, 18, 46, 65, 84
Catabolism, 131, 143
CATAPRES, 4, 55
CECLOR, 7, 57
Cefaclor, 24, 31, 32, 50, 69, 74, 75, 87
Cefazolin, 13, 61
Cefprozil, 18, 65
Cefuroxime, 48, 86
CELEBREX, 42, 82
Celecoxib, 12, 60

CELLCEPT, 26, 71
Cephalexin, 50, 87
Cerebellum, 134, 145
Cerebrospinal fluid, 131, 143
CEREBYX, 19, 66
CHF (congestive heart failure), 125, 139
Chloral hydrate, 30, 73
Chlorpropamide, 49, 86
Chondrodynia, 134, 145
Chronic bronchitis, 164, 181
CII (controlled drug class 2), 125, 139
Cimetidine, 27, 51, 71, 87
Ciprofloxacin, 7, 9, 13, 14, 41, 44, 57, 58, 61, 62, 81, 83
Cirrhosis, 163, 181
Clarithromycin, 19, 34, 47, 48, 66, 76, 85, 86
CLARITIN, 3, 8, 9, 11, 23, 54, 58, 59, 68, 159, 178
Class IV controlled substance, 204, 215
CLINORIL, 52, 88
Clomipramine, 47, 85
Clonazepam, 4, 5, 39, 50, 51, 55, 79, 87
Clonidine patches, 19, 66
CMV (cytomegalovirus), 126, 140
CNS (central nervous system), 132, 144
Codeine, 156, 176
Colchicine, 3, 9, 36, 50, 51, 54, 58, 77, 87, 88
COLESTID, 25, 70
COMBIVENT, 31, 74
Common ailments and drug treatments, 162–171
Commonly prescribed medications, 1–52
Congestive heart failure, 164; *see also* CHF
Conjugated estrogens, 24, 25, 35, 42, 46, 48, 69, 70, 77, 82, 84, 86
Constipation, 162, 163, 180
Controlled substance schedules, 204–205, 208
Conversions, 89–123
Convulsions, 164, 181
Copper sulfate, 33, 76
COREG, 10, 59
CORLOPAM, 32, 75
Corticosteroids, 33, 76
CORTISPORIN, 46, 84
CORVERT, 22, 68
Co-trimoxazole, 23, 69
COUMADIN, 2, 30, 53, 73
CRNA, 135, 146
Cyclopentolate, 162, 180
Cyclophosphamide, 14, 62
Cyclosporine, 21, 67
CYTOTEC, 14, 62
CYTOXAN, 7, 57

D

DARVOCET-N, 12, 61
DARVON, 207, 217

DAYPRO, 9, 58
DEA (Drug Enforcement Administration), 126, 140
Depression, 166, 183
Dermatitis, 127, 140
Desipramine, 19, 66
DESOWEN, 45, 84
DIABETA, 51, 87
Diarrhea, 162
Diclofenac, 8, 12, 16, 22, 26, 31, 37, 57, 60, 64, 68, 71, 74, 79
DIFLUCAN, 5, 56
Digibind, 36, 77
Digoxin, 21, 22, 26, 34, 37, 38, 39, 40, 67, 68, 71, 76, 78, 79, 80
Digoxin tablets, 39, 80
DILANTIN, 35, 77
Diltiazem, 13, 15, 26, 31, 33, 39, 44, 46, 62, 71, 74, 75, 76, 80, 83, 84
DIOVAN, 18, 65
Diphenhydramine, 5, 28, 46, 56, 72, 84
Diphenylhydantonin, 8, 58
Dispensing process, 148–186
Distribution, 187–194
Diuretics, 163, 180
Divalproex, 164, 181
DNR ("do not resuscitate"), 128, 141
Donepezil, 43, 82
Dopamine, 11, 38, 60, 79
Doxazosin, 35, 77
Doxycycline, 13, 61
Drug Facts and Comparisons, 203, 215
DT (delirium tremens), 132, 144
Duodenal ulcers, 37, 78
DURAGESIC patch, 206, 216
DYAZIDE, 9, 58
DYNACIRC, 42, 82
Dyspnea, 137, 147

E

Edema, 18, 65
Electronic and computer information, 195–209
Enalapril, 2, 8, 17, 19, 29, 39, 46, 53, 58, 65, 66, 72, 80, 85
Epilepsy, 162, 165, 180
Epinephrine, 22, 68, 154, 175
Epsom salt, 30, 73
Eptifibatide, 9, 59
Equipment, maintenance of, 195–209
Ergocalciferol, 36, 78
ERYTHROCIN, 137, 147
Erythrocyte, 132, 143
Erythromycin, 207, 217
Estradiol, 26, 70
Ethinyl estradiol/levonorgestrel, 3, 4, 6, 54, 55, 56
Etodolac, 18, 65
EULEXIN, 39, 80

F

Facilities, maintenance of, 195–209
Famotidine, 7, 20, 49, 50, 57, 66, 86, 87
FDA (Federal Drug Association), 203, 207, 215, 217
FELDENE, 52, 88
Fentanyl, 24, 29, 70, 73
FERGON, 51, 87
Fever, 163, 165, 182
FIORICET, 14, 62
FLEXERIL, 52, 88
FLONASE, 40, 81
Fluconazole, 24, 32, 33, 44, 49, 69, 75, 83, 86
Flumazenil, 27, 71
Fluoxetine, 2, 35, 41, 47, 53, 77, 81, 85
FOLOX, 38, 79
FOSAMAX, 11, 59
Furosemide, 4, 8, 11, 28, 29, 34, 51, 55, 58, 60, 72, 73, 76, 88

G

Gastric ulcers, 37, 78
Gastritis, 136, 146
Gastrointestinal, 130, 142
Gemfibrozil, 4, 38, 55, 79
Generic medications, 1–52
Genitourinary system, 129, 142
GERD (gastroesophageal reflux disease), 131, 143
Glassine paper, 158, 177
Glipizide, 13, 21, 33, 35, 40, 61, 67, 76, 77, 80
GLUCOPHAGE, 16, 64
GLUCOTROL, 5, 55
Glyburide, 10, 25, 26, 41, 42, 59, 70, 81, 82
Glycosuria, 127, 137, 140, 147
GLYSET, 125, 139
Gold sodium thiomalate, 27, 29, 33, 71, 73, 76

H

HALDOL, 163, 181
HCO$_3$, 133, 144
Helicobacter pylori, 160, 179
Hemapoiesis, 135, 146
Hematocyte, 129, 142
Heparin, 136, 146
Hepatic, 131, 143
Homeostasis, 134, 145
Human resources, roles, duties, and responsibilities, 195–209
HUMULIN, 2, 22, 53, 68
Hydrochloroquine, 42, 81
Hydrochlorothiazide, 20, 66
Hydrocortisone, 125, 139, 161, 180
Hydroxychloroquine, 6, 11, 28, 34, 35, 56, 60, 72, 77

Hyoscyamine, 25, 70
Hyperalimentation, 127, 140
Hyperemia, 135, 146
Hyperglycemic, 9, 59
Hyperlipidemia, 159, 178
Hypertension, 163, 180
Hypokalemic, 130, 143

I

Ibuprofen, 12, 30, 38, 60, 73, 79
Idoxuridine, 16, 63
IMODIUM, 19, 66
INDERAL, 50, 87
Indinavir, 28, 72
Insulin, 31, 32, 36, 37, 40, 74, 75, 78, 80, 125, 139
Insulin-dependent diabetes mellitus, 8, 58
Integumentary system, 129, 142
Intracranially, 137, 147
INTRALIPIDS, 35, 77
Inventory system, 187–194
Ipecac, 30, 73
Ipecac syrup, 45, 84
ISOPTIN, 20, 66
Isosorbide, 24, 69
Itraconazole, 38, 79
IV, preparation, 157, 177

J

Jargons, 124–147
JCAHO (Joint Commission on Accreditation of Health Care Organizations), 136, 147

K

KAY CIEL, 24, 50, 69, 87
K-CLOR, 46, 84
Ketamine, 24, 70, 205, 216
Ketoconazole, 51, 87
Ketoprofen, 37, 78
Ketorolac, 10, 15, 32, 37, 59, 63, 75, 78
KLONOPIN, 11, 60

L

Lamotrigine, 25, 70
LANOXIN, 31, 74
LASIX, 11, 60
Leukotrienes, 159, 178
LEVAQUIN, 20, 67
Levothyroxine, 2, 23, 25, 36, 45, 48, 53, 68, 70, 78, 84, 86
Lisinopril, 24, 33, 36, 48, 70, 76, 78, 85
Lithium, 24, 69, 134, 145
Liver, 131, 143
LOMOTIL, 32, 75
Loperamide, 17, 64, 162, 180
LOPRESSOR, 43, 83

Loratidine, 3, 9, 16, 43, 48, 54, 58, 64, 82, 86
Lorazepam, 49, 86
Lovastatin, 7, 32, 34, 41, 43, 56, 75, 76, 77, 81, 82
LOVENOX, 15, 63, 128, 141
Lungs, 130, 142
LUPRON, 42, 82

M

MAALOX, 131, 143
MACRODANTIN, 15, 44, 63, 83
Macrolide antibiotics, 22, 23, 30, 68, 69, 74
Magnesium, 133, 144
Malpractice, 204, 215
Management of facilities, 195–209
MAO inhibitors, 14, 21, 22, 27, 62, 67, 68, 71
Mastodynia, 135, 145
Mathematical calculations, 89–123
MAXALT, 10, 59
MAXIPIME, 9, 58
MAXZIDE, 4, 54, 166, 183
MDI (metered-dose inhaler), 132, 144
Medical abbreviations, 124–147
Medication orders, understanding and interpreting, 148–186
Medroxyprogesterone, 10, 12, 39, 44, 45, 59, 61, 80, 83, 84
MedWatch, 138, 147
MEGACE, 24, 49, 69, 86
Meperidine, 154, 175, 204, 215
Metformin, 12, 60
Methotrexate, 6, 27, 38, 56, 72, 79
Methylphenidate, 16, 64
Methylprednisolone, 33, 76
Metoclopramide, 38, 39, 79
Metoprolol, 28, 29, 72
Metronidazole, 8, 20, 22, 23, 30, 57, 58, 67, 68, 69, 74
MEVACOR, 16, 63
MICRONASE, 31, 74
Midazolam, 24, 70
MINIPRESS, 8, 43, 58, 82
Minocycline, 15, 29, 50, 63, 73, 87
Minoxidil, 20, 67
MOTRIN, 14, 62
MUCOMYST, 17, 64
Mupirocin, 47, 85
Myocardial infarctions, 165, 182

N

Nabumetone, 3, 33, 47, 54, 76, 85
Nafcillin, 21, 67
Naphazoline, 12, 61, 127, 140
NAPROSYN, 29, 72
Naproxen, 14, 21, 27, 28, 62, 68, 72
NASACORT, 52, 88

NASALCROM, 28, 52, 72, 88
National Association of Chain Drug Stores (NACDS), 203, 215
Nebulizer ("neb"), 125, 139
Nefzodone, 23, 69
NEORAL, 45, 84
NEOSPORIN, 17, 64
NEO-SYNEPHRINE, 12, 60
Nephrotoxicity, 128, 141
NEUPOGEN, 15, 63, 131, 143
NEURONTIN, 18, 65
Nifedipine, 5, 18, 21, 29, 49, 55, 65, 67, 73, 86
Nisoldipine, 42, 81
Nitroglycerin, 27, 71, 166, 182
Nizatidine, 3, 25, 26, 28, 29, 54, 70, 71, 72, 73
NORCO, 205, 216
NORFLEX, 46, 84
NORVASC, 7, 57
NSAIDs, 5, 55, 166, 183

O

Omeprazole, 3, 6, 18, 32, 34, 35, 41, 54, 56, 65, 75, 76, 77, 81
Ondansetron, 17, 21, 24, 65, 67, 70, 164, 181
Orange Book code, 203
Ordering, 187–194
Osteo, 130, 142
Osteoarthritis, 161, 179
Oxycodone, 9, 58, 205, 216

P

Paclitaxel, 6, 24, 30, 39, 45, 50, 56, 69, 73, 80, 83, 87
Pamidronate, 163, 181
Paroxetine, 20, 27, 31, 67, 71, 74
PAXIL, 11, 60
Penicillamine, 10, 59
Penicillin, 46, 84, 126, 134, 139, 145
Penicillin VK, 3, 5, 6, 54, 56
PEPCID, 21, 52, 67, 88
Pericarditis, 136, 147
Pericardium, 136, 146
PERMAX, 23, 69
Pharmaceutical abbreviations/acronyms, 124–147
Pharmaceutical calculations, 89–123
Pharmacokinetics, 158, 177
Pharmacy technician, duties of, 201
Phenazopyridine, 6, 56
Phenylbutazone, 19, 66
Phenytoin, 7, 17, 22, 26, 32, 34, 37, 40, 44, 48, 57, 64, 68, 71, 75, 77, 78, 80, 83, 85, 162, 180
Phytanodione, 13, 61
Piroxicam, 34, 47, 77, 85

PLAQUENIL, 4, 10, 55, 59
PLAVIX, 4, 5, 55
PLETAL, 133, 144
Policies and the retail sector, management of, 195–209
Potassium, 133, 145
Potassium chloride, 32, 38, 39, 41, 43, 75, 79, 80, 81, 83
Potassium-sparing diuretics, 33, 75
Pramipexole, 10, 59
Pravastatin, 4, 28, 42, 55, 72, 82
Prazosin, 25, 37, 42, 45, 47, 70, 79, 82, 84, 85
Pre-eclampsia, 129, 142
PREMARIN, 13, 61
Prescriptions, understanding and interpreting, 148–186
PRN, 126, 140
Procainamide, 27, 71
Product preparation, 148–186
Propofol, 36, 78
Propoxyphene, 30, 45, 48, 74, 84, 86
Prostate cancer, 39, 80
Protamine, 46, 85
Protease inhibitors, 43, 83
Protein anabolism, 161, 179
PROTONIX, 14, 62, 178
PROVERA, 12, 60
PROZAC, 5, 55, 131, 143
PTCA procedure, 137, 147
Purchasing, 187–194

Q

q2hprn schedule, 127, 140
Quetiapine, 13, 61
Quinidine, 21, 67
Quinine, 36, 78
Quinolone antibiotics, 20, 66

R

Ranitidine, 4, 34, 36, 37, 39, 40, 44, 48, 49, 55, 76, 78, 79, 80, 81, 83, 86
Records, maintenance of, 195–209
REFLAFEN, 9, 58
Regulations, standards, and ethics, 203–209
REMERON, 26, 70
Renal, 131, 143
Rheumatoid arthritis, 135, 146
Rhinitis, 127, 140
ROBINUL, 23, 44, 69, 83

ROBITUSSIN DAC, 152, 174
ROGAINE, 20, 67

S

Script, 149
SELSUN, 31, 74
SERAX, 134, 145
SEROQUEL, 130, 143
Sertraline, 3, 6, 23, 33, 40, 48, 53, 56, 68, 76, 80, 81, 85
Sickle cells, 132, 144
Silver sulfadiazine, 30, 43, 74, 82
Simvastatin, 3, 5, 6, 40, 44, 54, 56, 80, 83, 165, 182
SINEMET, 38, 79
SLOW-K, 19, 66
SMZ (sulfamethoxazole), 125, 139
Solution, 157, 177
SOMA COMPOUND, 41, 81
SSRI (Selective serotonin reuptake inhibitor), 2, 4, 15, 53, 63, 136, 146
State Board of Pharmacy, 205, 216
Steven-Johnson syndrome, 35, 77
Subpoena, 205, 216
Sulindac, 26, 71
Suspension, 157, 177
Symbols, medical/pharmaceutical, 124–147
SYMMETREL, 18, 26, 65, 70
SYNTHROID, 24, 69

T

Tachycardia, 136, 146
Tacrolimus, 27, 71
Tamoxifen, 2, 25, 53, 70
TAPAZOLE, 51, 87
Tavist-1, 28, 72
TAXOL, 5, 11, 55, 60
Temazepam, 50, 87
Terbutaline, 20, 66
Terminology, medical/pharmaceutical, 124–147
Tetracycline, 7, 57, 136, 147
Thalidomide, 15, 63
Theophylline, 7, 57
Thioridazine, 15, 62
Thiothixene, 30, 73
THORAZINE, 18, 65
TIAZAC, 130, 142
Timolol, 44, 83
TMP (trimethoprim), 125, 139

TOPROL XL, 41, 81
TORADOL, 2, 53
TRENTAL, 44, 83
Tretinoin, 166, 183
Triamterene/hydrochlorothiazide, 11, 60
Tricyclic antidepressants, 136, 146
TRIPHASIL 28, 8, 57
Tuberculin, 152, 174

U

ULTRAM, 12, 61
Urinary tract infection, 6, 56, 131, 143

V

VALIUM, 207, 217
VANTIN, 38, 79
Vasoconstrictor ("vaso"), 126, 140
VASOTEC, 34, 77
V-CILLIN K, 2, 53
Vecuronium, 29, 73
Venlafaxine, 43, 83
VENTOLIN, 50, 87
Verapamil, 2, 3, 4, 14, 16, 17, 53, 54, 62, 64
VERELAN, 15, 63
VERSED, 160, 178
VICODIN, 137, 147
VOLMAX, 50, 87
VOLTAREN, 10, 59

W

Warfarin, 7, 17, 20, 42, 47, 57, 65, 66, 67, 82, 85

X

XALATAN, 23, 69
XYLOCAINE, 25, 70

Z

ZANAFLEX, 12, 45, 60, 84
ZAROXYLYN, 10, 59
ZEBETA, 16, 17, 64
ZESTRIL, 7, 57
ZOFRAN, 9, 34, 58, 76
ZOLOFT, 19, 20, 65, 66, 67, 166, 183
ZOSYN, 27, 41, 71, 81
ZOVIRAX, 17, 64
Z-Pack, 40, 80
ZYPREXA, 13, 61, 163, 181